KU-825-928

Y

The Nursing Sister

By the same author

When Matron Ruled

The Nursing Sister

A Caring Tradition

PETER ARDERN

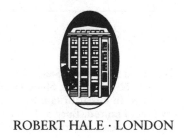

ROBERT HALE · LONDON

© Peter Ardern 2005
First published in Great Britain 2005

ISBN 0 7090 7415 8

Robert Hale Limited
Clerkenwell House
Clerkenwell Green
London EC1R 0HT

A catalogue record for this book is available from the British Library

2 4 6 8 10 9 7 5 3 1

Typeset in 9¾/12¾pt Sabon by
Derek Doyle & Associates, Shaw Heath.
Printed in Great Britain by
St Edmundsbury Press Limited, Bury St Edmunds, Suffolk.
Bound by Woolnough Bookbinding Limited.

To June

Contents

Acknowledgements

I would like to acknowledge the help and encouragement I have received from many people. The members of the NHS Retirement Association, Cosham, the 'Digger' historical group and Ursula Ward, Director of Nursing and Midwifery, Queen Alexandra Hospital, Portsmouth.

Once again a special thank you goes to Sharon Zak (née Thorpe) for her invaluable insights and judicious comments. In this respect thanks are also due to Ruth Sanders, Gary Standing, Mike Owen and Geoffrey Yeo, author of *Nursing at Bart's*.

Thanks must also go to the many people who gave up their time for interview, to those who loaned precious photographs, personal diaries and documents and to those who wish to remain anonymous. Thank you to Roy Stallard, who proved once again to be invaluable in contacts and material. To Alex Attewell and the staff at the Florence Nightingale Museum, Dorothy A. Hancock for information regarding Sister Elizabeth Hancock. To Pamela Fontana for information concerning Mary Potter and the Greene family for use of notes and diary from John's life. Also, to Derek Sykes and Peter Young (graphics department) Haslar Hospital.

Finally, a special thank you to my wife June for being a patient travel companion and secretary, to whom this book is dedicated.

List of Illustrations

Between pages 96 and 97

11

30   Clinical teacher Lynette Patterson at Queen Mary's Hospital for children, London, 1972
31   Sister Kay Riley leading daily prayers on Elizabeth Ward, St Thomas's Hospital, 1960
32   Sisters Janet Campbell and Seta Singh on the elderly care ward and in the uniform of South Western Hospital, London, 1979
33   Sister Ann Gross and Sister Denise Rock at Queen Alexandra Hospital, Cosham, following a weight-loss fund-raising event
34   Midwife Jennie Vinall, Matron Margaret Pettigrew, Avril Williamson   and, seated, Mrs Pettigrew at Blake House, Gosport, 1966
35   Dorothy Turner and Cynthia Braithwaite in nurse training at Bolingbroke Hospital, 1963
36   Sister Margaret Window gowned up to attend to a patient with TB meningitis at Rush Green Hospital, c. 1957
37   Tri-service nursing sisters, Lieutenant Maria Rea (Navy), Captain Lyndsey Hunter (Army), and Flight Lieutenant Helene Martin (Air Force) in traditional uniform, 2004

Credits

Foreword

From Florence Nightingale onwards the responsibilities placed on the nursing sister across a range of nursing disciplines have been increasing and the sister role has evolved accordingly. I am proud to have known and worked with many remarkable sisters, some of whom have dedicated their whole lives to nursing. They have been the backbone of hospital life and have played their parts in the success of our modern health service.

In this book, memories will be evoked of the years when sisters were involved in giving attention to every detail on their wards or wherever they worked in the community. High standards were expected from everyone and in this respect the sister led from the front by example. Sticklers for cleanliness, they were hands-on.

Major changes have occurred across our hospitals and nursing services since the time of Nightingale: two world wars, the introduction of the National Health Service, the demise of the matron as head of nursing, reorganizations and the introduction of the modern matron. Throughout all these changes the role of the sister has been consistent and central to the continuing success of the health service.

As matron of a large teaching hospital in Manchester, I personally knew the value of ward sisters; I promoted most of them. Having come through the same training system I knew their work and their capabilities, and respected them for their expertise. The sisters were promoted on merit, having proved their worth and had earned the post by the time they were advanced. They had worked alongside experienced sisters and spent time in an acting post gaining invaluable knowledge.

We all lived in, in my day. Living in the nurses' home gave us a sense of comradeship that has lasted many years. Looked after by 'fussy', caring home sisters and sister tutor, we would work hard and at times play hard too. There were no discos, of course; could you imagine a matron at that time permitting them? But we did manage to escape the long hours and stresses of nursing through more temperate but no less enjoyable activities.

A lot of our time was spent at the bedside. I still recall the words of Sister Dawson when I was a junior nurse: 'I can teach you all about nursing but I cannot teach you common sense, young lady.' Those sisters taught us a great deal; they were at the bedside and taught by example. A lot of nursing is about common sense, even today: ensuring that patients are able to feed themselves, ensuring that hands are washed, making sure the ward area is clean and patients are able to relate to someone clearly in authority on a daily basis. Common sense coupled with nursing expertise is a pretty powerful combination.

We should not live in the past, the clock cannot be turned back and some of the old days I would not wish back. But we should not ignore the past either. Now retired, I can spend time looking back and see what a wonderful training we had. It was mainly on the wards gaining practical experience with patients under the ever-watchful eye and tutorship of the ward sister. I can only hope that sisters now are able to maintain this role and avoid the ever-present danger of finding themselves in an administrative role where they may lose clinical contact with the patients and training opportunities with the nurses.

Standards and values have always been upheld vigorously by sisters – too vigorously some might argue – but unifying standards and promoting values were seen as important. There are complaints that there is less respect now, and that the constant demands on sisters from every direction are very trying. Expectations are higher and the throughput of patients much faster, so it is more important than ever that sisters are able to maintain their position as upholders of nursing standards.

Clarice Bell
Former matron of Manchester Royal Infirmary

14

1 The Sisterhoods

If a religious head of a religious order has undivided authority over a hospital it will be badly nursed. If a medical staff has individual authority over hospital nursing the hospital will be badly nursed. Otherwise, it matters not whether the nurses are lay-women, Anglican or any other 'sisters', nuns or what not, the one essential thing is that they be trained good nurses . . .
Florence Nightingale, letter to Harry Bonham-Carter, 1866

To understand the traditional role of our nursing sisters it is important that we briefly explore the early history of these remarkable post-holders. This chapter explains the role of the religious orders, many of which were the forerunners of our modern sisters. They provided what little organized nursing there was in the centuries leading up to the Florence Nightingale revolution in hospital organization and nurse training. These were the orders where the title 'Sister' originated.

In *How to Become a Nurse*, written in about 1925, M.E. Fox wrote:

Sooner or later, almost every girl has a desire to become a nurse. It may be because she wishes to do some good in the world; to be independent; to have a career; perhaps, because she is tired of her present occupation and desires a change; or it may be for the simple reason that she is obliged by force of circumstances, to make her own way in the world and thinks she may as well earn her living in a hospital as anywhere else. Not every girl, of course, who takes up nursing does so because she likes, above all things, to look after sick people. When this does happen, she is that *rara avis* – a 'born nurse'.

15

This extract reflects society's limited attitude towards aspiring young ladies at the time. Limited in any professional opportunities, women were still in the main offered a life in service – service to one's God, the sick, a mistress in a household or a husband. Nursing presented a challenging and radical alternative, a career – a career regarded as respectable for women, something unthinkable eighty years earlier when Charles Dickens portrayed the characters of Sairey Gamp and Betsy Prig to reflect his 'reformist' view of nursing for the poor sick. Dickens wrote that Mrs Sairey Gamp was a fair representation of the hired attendant on the poor in the community and that Mrs Betsy Prig was a fair specimen of a St Bartholomew's Hospital nurse.

Before this infamous pair graced the pages of *Martin Chuzzlewit*, religion and nursing had been closely linked. The monasteries were the places where the poor sick could find some care, with monks and nuns being the only people recognized as practising medicine and nursing. Outside the monasteries women (wisewomen) were predominantly the healers for the poor, with the few male counterparts practising the new profession of medicine and surgery at the courts in London, the military services, and for the more affluent in society.

The three main medieval hospitals of St Bartholomew's, St Thomas's and Bedlam were religious foundations whose principal object was to provide a comfortable environment for the sick poor in the hope that rest, regular meals, and constant prayer would alleviate their suffering. These institutions were small and only provided accommodation for a tiny proportion of those in need. Society as a whole had neither the skill nor the inclination to improve the conditions of these people.

Throughout the monastic period, members of the Augustinian order were the 'nurses'. They entered the order for the contemplation of a religious life, to serve God and to care for the sick. The Reformation, beginning in 1534 in this country, sounded the death knell for many poor sick as it swept away monastic life, including the few hospitals there were. The only survivor was St Bartholomew's Hospital, London. For the poor sick this was such a calamity that King Henry VIII was finally compelled to re-found St Thomas's Hospital in 1550. This change precipitated the emergence of a role for the ward sister. Their role simply entailed supplying practical daily living needs; their duties were to keep the patients clean, give them regular food, make their beds and wash their clothes.

One of the oldest and most important nursing orders of nuns working under a strictly monastic system was based at the Hôtel Dieu on the River Seine in Paris, a hospital for the poor sick founded by Landry, the Bishop of Paris. Those in the order, which dated back to the twelfth century, were vowed to poverty, chastity, and obedience. Known as 'sisters', the nurses of this Augustinian order, founded under the Rule of St Augustine AD 650, served God by extreme hard work. In pious dedication they set to all manner of household work, even washing soiled linen in the River Seine, breaking the ice in the depths of winter to complete their task. The sisters undertook a long probationary period, first becoming a 'white sister', and many years later receiving the hood of a 'chaperon sister'. Unusual for the time, these sisters were often in charge of male wards, with the religious brothers working for them.

For its period the Hôtel Dieu was a beacon of care for the poor sick throughout Europe, but compared even to the time when Florence Nightingale began her reforms, the conditions in which the patients were nursed were extremely primitive. Nevertheless the dedication of these sisters is without parallel, and they have provided a continuous service for over twelve centuries, the longest nursing service by any religious order. The Hôtel Dieu accommodated well over a thousand patients, distributed between twenty-five wards.

A sixteenth-century priest wrote of the Hotel Dieu that it had little consideration for the need for fresh air, space between beds or general hygiene. In a bed would be six sick patients, the feet of one next to the head of another, children next to old people, men next to women. In the same bed lay people who had infectious diseases next to people only slightly unwell. Women could be in childbirth next to a typhus sufferer. The most miserable food was given out in tiny quantities and not at regular intervals, but anyone could bring anything in. So while the sick might starve one day, the next day they might get drunk and kill themselves by overloading their stomachs. The whole building swarmed with rats, and the air was so vile in the sick wards that the attendants did not enter without a sponge soaked in vinegar held to their face. The bodies of the dead often lay in bed for more than a day. It was with a mixture of faith and hope that patients recovered from the simplest of surgical operations – there being only one surgeon. The hospital had no designated operating theatre and only five surgical instruments, which included a trephine for opening the skull and a mouth plug for keeping the jaws separated. The sisters' working day was directed by the priests not the doctors, and it was not considered suitable that celibate nuns should know about, let alone see, the patients' bodies. In the middle of the seventeenth century the French priest Vincent de Paul took a timely and extremely practical interest when visiting the hospital. Through him the obedience of the sisters was shifted from the priests to the physicians. It needed to be.

By the nineteenth century Germany had the Kaiserswerth Deaconesses' Institution near Düsseldorf. In 1822, the young Lutheran Theodor Fliedner saw so much sickness and suffering among his poor parishioners that he set about collecting funds to provide care. With this money he built an institution that provided high-quality nurse training to the deaconesses. Both the institution and the deaconesses were to receive recognition throughout the western world. Such was its reputation that Florence Nightingale spent time there herself learning about nursing.

In England, Mrs Elizabeth Gurney Fry was greatly influenced by the work of the Kaiserswerth Institution. In the 1800s nurses were widely regarded with suspicion and contempt by the general population. Hospitals were beginning to open throughout the country following the ravages of the Reformation, but care was basic and often relied on goodwill rather than good nursing. For poor sick individuals in the community little had changed. Mrs Fry set about changing that perception by instructing her nurses as thoroughly as the knowledge and circumstances of the time permitted. Quite radically, she arranged for nurses to attend a general hospital for instruction every day during their training. This mighty act was recognized as a considerable advancement in nurse training. Mrs Fry, being a most benevolent and far-sighted woman, inaugurated the Protestant Institute of Nursing Sisters in 1840. Recognizing the necessity for providing more nurses in private homes Mrs Fry's idea was to supply nurses of character and efficiency who would become skilled and trustworthy attendants for the sick.

The usefulness and dependability of these pioneer private nurses led to the formation of a scheme at St John's House, London, for the better nursing of hospital patients. This initiative, in turn, further developed the quality and availability of private nurses for the wealthy sick. Inaugurated in 1848, St John's House was a community of sisters who, with the support of King's College Hospital, trained nurses to attend the sick. At King's College there was a newly defined icon, the matron, under whom came sisters, whose work was unpaid. Nurses, on the other hand, were trained and paid for their work. King's College Hospital continued with the tradition of naming the matron, Sister Matron, in line with its religious origins well into the 1950s; Sister Matron Eve Opie was the last to be known by this title when she retired. Ward sisters at this hospital also maintained the links with the past; they were known by Christian names, but not their own names. When a nurse was promoted to sister, she would choose a name from a specific list, like the nuns in the religious orders of old.

The sisters were deemed to be ladies of higher birth or church-women of impeccable character, who performed their duties as an act of religious commitment and service to the sisterhood. The trainee nurses were drawn from a lower social class. All candidates for training had to furnish certificates of baptism into the Church of England. Trained under the sisters the nurses knew their work thoroughly, having had one year's training before being admitted. The Lady Superintendent of St John's House allotted the work, ensuring that it was appropriate to the grade. In 1870 she wrote: 'In this arrangement, St John's House was in advance of its time, but the auxiliary departments of the hospital (the departments of the kitchen, linen, and bedding supplies) are now regarded as forming an integral part of nursing as scientifically understood.' For many years, the sisters headed these departments.

Until the end of the nineteenth century the University College Hospital of London was nursed almost entirely by the sisters of All Saints Church. In 1859, the Mother Foundress of the All Saints Sisterhood, Miss Brownlow-Byron, asked for two of her nurses to attend University College Hospital for the purpose of learning to nurse the sick and wounded. These sisters, and others who helped in the hospital, were held in the highest regard by medical staff, who were pleased not only by their disciplined, quiet and sedate appearance, but also by the impact they had on the cleanliness of the wards and the patients. The staff consisted of a head sister who acted as lady superintendent and one head nurse (sister) for every two wards. They were all directly responsible to the Mother Superior of All Saints. These sisters had a beneficial effect on the wards, with the level of drunkenness and theft falling considerably. This arrangement continued until 1898 when it was found that, good as the nursing was, the lady superintendent did not manage the accounting system quite so well. The contract between the All Saints Sisters and University College Hospital was ended, with a secular matron and sisters appointed in their place.

In 1847, Miss Priscilla Lydia Sellon moved to Devonport and quickly began recruiting the first sisters to her new Anglican Sellonite order. Although she was a woman of modest means, with the support of these sisters she purchased three large houses in the slums of Plymouth. Through the two cholera outbreaks of 1849 and 1852 they not only excelled at nursing sick patients, but they had also built a small hospital to admit the worst cases. The order grew and eventually acquired a base in London by amalgamating with the St Saviour's Sisterhood. This order provided eight sisters for the Florence Nightingale nursing group in the Crimea, beginning their work at Scutari Hospital in 1854.

In Ireland at this time, Nana Nagle, Catherine MacAuley and Mary Aikenhead were among a number of religious sisters taking an interest in the sick poor. The living conditions and the disturbing levels of disease in Dublin, where typhus and cholera were rife, appalled them. Sister Mary Aikenhead founded the Irish Sisterhood of Charity. Her aims were simple and modest, merely to help the sick and poor in their own homes. The order quickly grew and became well known throughout the counties bordering Dublin. Not trained as nurses, they struggled to deal with diseases like typhus, cholera and tuberculosis. Sister Aikenhead, the first Mother Superior, acknowledged this shortcoming and arranged for some of the sisters to be trained in Paris. This led to the opening of St Vincent's Hospital, Dublin, a hospital Miss Nightingale always held in high regard. To this day the sisters are remembered for their exacting standards of hygiene, their diligence in carrying out nursing duties, and their care of the sick. A wealthy woman, Miss Aikenhead, like the other religious sisters, was constantly constrained by the bishopric, but through determination and often with the use of subterfuge they managed to circumscribe an endless number of obstacles.

Another pioneer was Mary Potter. Born in London in 1847, she soon experienced the pain of a broken home. Moving with the family to Brighton and Portsmouth she had an overwhelming desire to follow a religious life, and entered the Convent of Mercy in Brighton at the age of twenty-one. At the age of twenty-nine she left and suffered throughout her life with heart disease and cancer. Having both breasts removed under minimal anaesthetic as a result of her heart condition, she understood the suffering of illness. After eight years of devotion to prayer for the sick and dying she developed the idea of opening a home to care for the most needy. Her brother George brought her idea to the attention of Bishop Bagshawe of Nottingham. In 1877, the bishop gave Mary permission to commence her work and sent her to Hyson Green. The convent, which also served as a mission chapel, was officially opened as the order of the Little Company of Mary by the bishop on Easter Monday 1877. Mary was not a woman of independent means so life was not easy; the sisters slept on straw and on occasions had very little to eat.

Although not a trained nurse herself, Mary recruited four other sisters, and these five ladies received the habit in 1877. They wore distinctive pale blue veils, by virtue of which they became commonly known as the 'blue nuns'. One of the recriuts was Sister Philip (formerly Edith Coleridge), who had trained at St George's Hospital, London. She and Mary taught the others the basics of hygiene and nursing, and they quickly became skilled in the care of the sick. Remarkably, Bishop Bagshawe allowed the sisters to become involved in midwifery care. In the late nineteenth century, when the incidence of infant and maternal mortality was excessively high, there was a great need for this type of provision. But the Church would not countenance it; it did not permit religious women to deliver babies, so this aspect of their work was stopped.

In the process of obtaining Vatican approval for the constitution of the order of the Little Company of Mary Sisters, Mother Mary Potter made several journeys to Rome, and consent was finally granted on 24 April 1893. At the time of approval the congregation had established houses in Italy, Ireland, Australia and America, and within twenty years there were sixteen houses. In addition a nurse training school had been opened in Limerick and they were caring for the sick in their own hospitals in Dublin and Galway.

Compassion, faith and Christian values travelled further than nursing the poor; they transcended boundaries. For example, many British soldiers readily recognized that they would not have survived the dreadful injuries they suffered in the Second World War had it not been for the intervention of sisterhoods in Germany. The Catholic Sisters of St Vincent were one notable group of nuns who time and time again helped allied servicemen. To them, human sympathy and care did not have boundaries.

Apart from the religious houses, the other group of women who became involved in caring for the sick were ladies of good family. Inspired by Christian charity, a desire to help the less fortunate or aspirations of independence and an urge to forge their own careers, they took to visiting the sick at home, as hospitals were not yet suitable places for such ladies. Although many of them went on to do great things in their careers, for example taking high-status positions as Nightingale's matrons and sisters, they were later criticized for being too prudish about physical care.

The conditions in many hospitals at the time were truly dreadful. As a result, most people avoided them if they could. Only the extremely ill or unconscious would submit to the dubious skills of the nursing profession. Of the rest, the better off employed private nurses and the poor fended for themselves, often dying untended in the slums where they lived, or had visits from the likes of Sairey Gamp. Dickens wrote about her as part of a reformist agenda in order to highlight the type of person employed as a professional nurse in the middle of the nineteenth century. In his descriptions of her he emphasized her drunkenness.

> She was a fat old woman, this Mrs. Gamp, with a husky voice and a moist eye, which she had a remarkable power of turning up, and only showing the white of. Having very little neck, it cost her some trouble to look over herself, if one may say so at those to whom she talked . . . The face of Mrs Gamp – the nose in particular – was somewhat red and swollen, and it was diffi-

cult to enjoy her society without becoming conscious of a smell of spirits. Like most persons who have attained to great eminence in the profession [nursing], she took to hers very kindly; insomuch, that setting aside her natural predilections as a woman, she went to a lying-in or a laying-out with equal zest and relish.

Her drinking habits, Dickens described as 'a pint of mild porter for lunch, a pint at dinner, half a pint as a species of stay or holdfast between dinner and tea, and a pint of the celebrated staggering ale, or Real Old Brighton Tipper, at supper; beside the bottle on the chimney-piece and other casual opportunities from "employers".'

This is a harsh description, and somewhat unfair to the many women who provided care to the sick, the sisterhoods. But other than these, all that was provided in the community and the hospitals amounted to little more than a specialized form of domestic service.

Drunkenness was an easy instrument with which to castigate the newly emerging 'profession' of nursing, but it has to be borne in mind that many nurses were actually paid in ale and with no running tap water, it was the safest thing to drink. Throughout the working population, from the dockyards to the newly emerging industries, drink was a problem. People were introduced to some form of alcohol early in life. When Thomas Hughes, the author of *Tom Brown's School Days*, was boarded at Rugby in the 1830s the boys almost only drank small beer (a weak beer). Fermented, it was a form of disease-free drink, in the absence of clean water.

In 1857 *The Times* did come to the defence of nurses, commenting:

Hospital nurses have been much abused – they have their faults, but most of them are due to want of proper treatment. Lectured by Committees, preached at by chaplains, scowled on by treasurers and stewards, scolded by matrons, sworn at by surgeons, bullied by dressers, grumbled at and abused by patients, insulted if old and ill-favoured, talked flippantly to if young and well-looking, they are what any woman might be under these circumstances.

There was also great confusion as to what constituted nursing and what were the tasks of the doctors, but quite clearly it was the latter who were the authority on the wards. It was they who changed dressings, applied poultices, gave enemas and amended dietary instructions. The taking of temperatures, pulses and blood pressures was not a routine activity for either doctors or nurses, and hardly anything would be charted. To compound the incompetence, many of the nurses were illiterate and would confuse prescribed instructions.

But the problem of drink was particularly difficult to overcome. Sister Casualty, a nurse at St Bartholomew's Hospital, wrote in 1902 about the time she began her training in 1877:

> Drunkenness was very common among the staff nurses, who were chiefly women of the charwoman type, frequently of bad character, with little or no education and few of them with even an elementary knowledge of nursing. Some of them might have worked previously at some other hospital but as often as not, they had no experience of nursing when they were engaged as 'staff' nurses. One woman, I remember, who came some little time after I did and under whom I worked, had been a lady's maid and had never done a day's nursing. She was, however, of a decidedly superior class to any of the others and was, moreover, quite respectable.

In addition to inferior quality nursing the need for ventilation was virtually unknown until Florence Nightingale began her hospital reforms. Windows at many hospitals were nailed shut. Damp, mildew and fungus flourished in the stagnant, moist atmosphere, as did a host of unsavoury creatures such as cockroaches, bed bugs and fleas. For the patients to be literally crawling with vermin was accepted as commonplace. Malnourished and dehydrated as the patients were, diseases spread easily from one to another and often to the nurses. Nurses scrubbed, laundered and emptied foetid spittoons and bedpans without the remotest semblance of sanitary systems. So it is not surprising that anyone with the least likelihood of getting better avoided these places, even to the extent of being left with crippling disabilities.

If conditions in the hospitals were less than satisfactory, the homes of the poor were often far worse. In Liverpool in the middle of the nineteenth century there were an estimated 38,000 people, out of a population of 250,000, living in cellars. It was not unusual for a family of five or more to be found living in one tiny cellar, and for three or four pigs to be sharing the same space. Fortunately the Industrial Revolution bought massive social changes. It needed healthy, fit workers. People who became ill through exposure to raw sewage in the streets and infested houses threatened the success of the rapidly developing industries. Hence there were sound economic reasons for introducing the first Public Health Act.

But a National Health Service was still many years away, and in the mean time nurses were also living in very poor conditions in the hospitals. This period of nursing has been called the 'Dark Age'. It was to be a major conflagration in southern Ukraine, the Crimea War, which was to act as the catalyst for changes that would spread to the hospital services.

It was during this war that Miss Florence Nightingale, with the title Superintendent of the Female Nursing Establishment of the English General Military Hospitals in Turkey, led a party of nurses who landed on the eastern shore of the Bosphorus. Among the group were upwards of fifty nurses from the various Anglican and Roman Catholic sisterhoods, many of whom proved to be the most successful nurses in the Crimea.

The soldiers in this war suffered appalling conditions in the hospitals, with disease killing more than the battles. Wounds would become so severely infected that the likelihood of survival was slim. So profound was the effect on Miss Nightingale that on her return to England in 1856 she set about reforming hospital administration, hygiene and nurse training. With these improvements and major developments in medical care, the service now needed more highly trained nurses.

2   Nightingale's Sisters

The whole reform in nursing both at home and abroad has
consisted in this: all power over the nursing out of the hands of
the men, and put it into the hands of one female trained head,
and make her responsible for everything (regarding internal
management and discipline) being carried out . . .

Florence Nightingale, letter to Mary Jones, Matron of
King's College Hospital, in 1867

Since the middle of the sixteenth century, the title 'sister' had designated the person who was head of the ward. The untrained hospital
sisters of these earlier centuries had been expected to undertake all
day-to-day 'domestic' work. Floors were strewn with rushes, patients
lay on straw mattresses, which were only burned when they were too
soiled to use. The ward sister transported all the coal, food and drink
to the wards. She emptied the slops, did the cleaning and even white-
washed the walls. She also washed all the patients' clothing and bed
linen.

By the middle of the seventeenth century the first simple hierarchical structure was in operation in the leading hospitals. It was
headed by a triad of medical officer, governor and matron, then came
sisters, nurses, helpers, maids and scrubbers. But it was not until the
eighteenth century that matrons' duties and responsibilities were
more clearly defined. They had to take charge of the household
goods and furniture and ensure the cleanliness of the bedchambers,
beds, clothes, linen and all things within the hospital. They would
visit the wards and offices daily to see that the sisters, nurses, helpers
and patients were observing the rules and doing their duty. In co-
operation with the ward sisters they would also ensure that the diets

for patients were correct.

On 1 June 1860, the following advertisement was placed in *The Times*:

The Nightingale Fund
To women desirous of being Trained as Hospital Nurses

The Committee of the Nightingale Fund have made
arrangements with the Authorities of St Thomas's Hospital for
giving a year's training to women, between 25 and 35 years of
age, for whom they will provide, free of expense, board and
lodging in the Hospital, with tea, sugar, and washing, and a
certain amount of outer clothing. A payment will be allowed
them of £10 for the year. They will be under the charge of the
Matron, and will be recommended for situations as hospital
nurses. The first quarter will commence on the 24th inst. For
further particulars apply to Mrs. Wardroper, St. Thomas's
Hospital. S.E., to whom all applications for admission must be
made.

Counsil Office, Downing Street, S.W.
A.H. Clough, Sec.

Arthur Hugh Clough, remembered for his romantic sea poetry, drafted this advertisement when he was first secretary of the Nightingale Fund and it heralded a major change in the quality of nurse applicant. Prior to the advent of Florence Nightingale's reforms, ward sisters gained their nursing experience in hospitals over many years working with the doctors, and were essentially there to carry out instructions. Any previous nursing experience was considered helpful but not essential for promotion to ward sister and it was only towards the end of the nineteenth century that the majority of sisters were promoted from the nursing staff.

The longest line of sisters, dating back to Sister Emma Charbury in the fifteenth century, was to be found at St Bartholomew's Hospital. For many years it had been the practice to recruit sisters from among respectable women who had experience of household work, who had been upper servants in private families or had been engaged to nurse the sick in their own homes. Occasionally the post was filled by one of the 'ordinary' nurses whose promotion was merited from length of service and assumed suitability. From this group came very many fine sisters, such as Mary Owen, Sister of Rahere Ward, St Bartholomew's Hospital, who was greatly respected. She was said to have carried out her work in an excellent manner for thirty-nine years, faithfully and kindly discharging her duties as nurse and sister. She bequeathed the sum of £250 to the hospital, remarkably, money she had saved from what must have been paltry earnings. Sisters in the large London hospitals were still earning only 18 shillings a week. This was a great improvement in every respect from the days when patients were charged by the sister one shilling on admission to her ward to supplement her wages of just a few shillings a month. These ward sisters could carry on working into their seventies and eighties.

As early as 1819 sisters at St Thomas's Hospital had been given clear instructions about their duties in respect of the administration of medicines. The sister was carefully to place all medicines for outward applications distinct from those for internal use, and to administer to the patients under their care the medicines prescribed by the physicians and surgeons of the hospital or delivered to them by the apothecary for that purpose. When called upon, she was to be ready to acquaint the physicians, surgeons or apothecary, with the effects of those medicines during their absence. She was to attend the apothecary's shop punctually to receive the medicines, taking great care that the labels or directions did not get lost or misplaced.

By 1870 the majority of hospitals had a sister as head of their wards. They now supervised the work of nurses in the care of the sick. Cleanliness in the ward and the maintenance of a good diet for patients were now paramount. In addition to the care of the sick, they had charge of the ward stores. They were now clearly the medium of communication between the patients and the medical staff, no longer the handmaidens for the doctors.

When St Thomas's Hospital was still in Surrey Gardens, one sister was in charge of eighty-eight beds. Each ward had one day nurse, two assistants and scrubbers, and one of the scrubbers acted as sister's maid. There was also one unsupervised night nurse. The work of these sisters remained for the most part menial for many years; they supervised, and in many cases engaged, in the cleaning of the wards. In addition, they were to be faithful and charitable at all times in attending the poor sick. Although there was no requirement to be trained in nursing skills they were expected to instruct their untrained helpers. However, much of the time was spent cleaning and sewing, a tradition of domesticity in nursing that seems to have continued unabated into relatively recent times. Lesley Smith remembers commencing her nurse training at Herrison Hospital, Dorset, in the 1930s. 'I spent most of my time on the day shifts cleaning, and most of my time on the night shifts with a needle in my hand.'

After Florence Nightingale's experiences in the Crimean War, and to counter the fragmentation of nurse training throughout the country, she began training nurses at the Nightingale School of Nursing, St Thomas's Hospital, London, in 1860 (shortly after her book, *Notes on Nursing* was published). The graduates of the school were known as 'Nightingales', and with their advent nursing as we know it began.

The school was funded by donations and the first matron was Mrs Wardroper. The probation nurses spent one year in training, living in private rooms with a common social room. At its height there were twenty to thirty pupils in a class. The school had two kinds of probationer. There were ladies of the higher social class with a superior education, who could purchase the opportunity to train; many of them went on to be the new matrons and ward sisters. Then there was the 'common class', who received expenses plus a small amount of money on completion of training. Some of them might rise to the rank of sister.

There were three basic principles for all hospitals which Miss Nightingale set out on the opening of her training school in 1860:

1 A trained matron was to be employed who had undisputed authority over all members of staff as well as probationer nurses.
2 A planned course of theoretical and practical training was to be given at the hospital to which the school was attached.
3 A nurses' home was to be established at every hospital and

carefully selected probationers were to be placed under the care of a sister specially chosen to be responsible for the moral and spiritual character training of the young women.

These new nurses began to enjoy a much higher status than their predecessors, but unfortunately remained at the mercy of ward sistersa of the old regime who could exercise whatever control they wished. These sisters had gained their knowledge of nursing through working closely with the doctors, and consequently could regulate the amount of knowledge passed on to the nurses. These new nurses could therefore easily be undermined.

During their training the probationer nurses were required to keep a diary and record special cases of disease, injury and operations, any other changes in a patient's condition, and any daily alterations in the management. This was the beginning of an enduring process of record-keeping in nursing. Besides the diaries each probationer would keep copious notes of the lectures they attended. Instruction was also given in the taking of pulse, temperature and respiration and how to give hypodermic injections. Very few nurses had previously been allowed to do these procedures; traditionally they were the duties of the junior medical staff. On the wards they worked very long hours and carried out duties that included as much cleaning as nursing.

In 1890 a 'special' probationer provided the following record of her day at St Thomas's Hospital. She rose at 6 a.m. and breakfasted at 6.30, ready to be on the ward by 7.a.m. She was detailed by ward sister to help on the night nurse side (the two sides of the ward were known, until modern times, as the night and day nurse sides), where she washed two patients. At 7.30 she helped on the day nurse side and washed a convalescent patient. At 8.00 she went to prayers in the chapel, then commenced washing a typhoid patient at 8.15. She commenced washing the urine bottles and the locker tops with chlorinated soda. From 8.45 she washed and dusted the sister's table and the window ledges, cleaned and trimmed the lamps, washed the urine and medicine glasses, small jugs and other ward apparel, prepared the lunch – bread and milk – and served it round to the patients. At 9.45 she went to the bathroom, where she washed out the bath, basins and traps. She put fresh cloths on the ice bowls, folded and put away the clean mattresses and tidied the pillow basket. She went off duty at 10.15, and at 11.00 had to attend the sister's class. She went to dinner at 12.45 p.m.

She came back on duty at 1.30, made beds with another nurse, washed the wine-glasses and dusted and tidied the centre of the ward. She put ready the dressing gowns for the doctor. At 1.50 she cut up 7 pounds of beef and made beef tea. At 2.20 she attended the doctor's round and waited on the sister. At 3.15 she went to the Steward's Office with a telegraphic message, and at 3.30 she helped the sister to wash an unconscious patient. She filled three steam kettles. At 4.20 she cut thin bread and butter for fever patients, prepared tea and served it round, and fed a patient. She went off duty 5.50. At 6.15 she was back on the ward, where she washed specimen glasses, feeders, and gas gloves, and gave the patients their supper. She made beds with another nurse. At 7.45 she tidied the centre of the ward and arranged and lit the lamps. She arranged the sister's desk and inkstand, took out the flowers and turned down the gas. At 8.00 she carried round the wines and brandy, at 8.15 collected the wine-glasses and at 8.30 went off duty. At 8.45 she went to prayers, at 9.00 had supper, and at 9.20 went to bed.

From the start, the fallout rate from the Nightingale School was very high. She thought that it must be a problem of selection, and in consultation with Mrs Wardroper, Miss Nightingale became more closely involved with choosing the probationers. It was at this point that she began to realize that the 'problem' was with the style of discipline, the long hours and the arduous work. All in all the life of a probationer was too harsh, and many of the probationers did not like being so closely supervised by the ward sisters; they expected to be treated more responsibly. They were accused of flirting if they even raised their eyes in male company; at least one nurse caused Mrs Wardroper and Miss Nightingale to exchange a flurry of correspondence about this problem. They were not allowed to 'chatter' as this was considered to be idle gossip. Even their off-duty attire was scrutinized before they were allowed out and even then were only allowed out of the hospital in pairs. This caused Miss Nightingale great consternation as she lived to the highest standards herself, and had expected her nurses to accept nothing less.

31

On completion of training, each nurse was expected to make the following pledge:

Florence Nightingale
Pledge to Nurses

I solemnly pledge myself before God and in the presence of this assembly to pass my life in purity and to practise my profession faithfully.

I will abstain from whatever is deleterious and mischievous, and will not knowingly administer any harmful drug.

I will do all in my power to elevate the standard of my Profession, and will hold in confidence all personal matters committed to my keeping, and all family affairs coming to my knowledge in the practice of my calling.

With loyalty will I endeavour to aid the Physician in his work, and devote myself to the welfare of those committed to my care.

This, I give to you, to guide you throughout your future years in this dedicated profession.

This moral exactitude demanded equally high moral standards and woe betide a nurse who faltered. Sister Elisabeth Hancock was one such. Dorothy A. Hancock writes that her great aunt trained at the Nightingale School at the end of the nineteenth century and signed the usual agreement that pupils would accept any placement that the school committee saw fit for a period of three years. Elisabeth was sent, along with a number of other pupils, to Edinburgh Royal Infirmary. During this placement she had an affair with one of the doctors and became pregnant. At that time it was unthinkable that a doctor should marry a nurse under any circumstances. It is not known how she coped but she managed to continue working as a sister. It was thought that her own sisters in London cared for the child (a boy).

One bitterly cold winter's night when Elisabeth was on duty, the fire needed fuelling. No porter being available she chose to go outside and fill the coal buckets. As a direct result of this she caught a chill and died. Following her death there was still no forgiveness for her or her son. At a time when the strict moral climate looked upon illegitimacy as a disgrace, her sisters decided that they and their nephew should emigrate to Australia. There was an assumption that the other members of the family did not know about Elisabeth's illegitimate son. Many years later Dorothy Hancock's Uncle Harry remembered a young man coming to the house when he was still a boy. Harry's father let the young man in but it was not long before he left again. When Harry enquired of his mother who the man was, he was told never to speak of it again. It was hard for Dorothy not to conclude that the young man must have been Sister Elisabeth's illegitimate son. She expressed sadness that this uncle could not forget the disgrace and accept him.

Along with the improvement in nursing heralded by the newly emerging structure, society was beginning to see hospitals as places where people could be cured, not just warehoused. Nevertheless some of the traditional problems were proving difficult to eradicate; there was a remarkable and disappointingly slow take-up of the Nightingale training programme at many of the London training hospitals, and it was even slower in the provincial hospitals until well into the 1880s.

Drunkenness was still common among nurses. 'Small beer' was openly provided and Lady Palmerston, like many in her time, did not think it wrong for nurses to drink on duty. By now they were allowed one pint or a pint and a half of strong porter daily, with one or two glasses of gin for disagreeable work such as laying out the dead, or for more repugnant work such as clearing infested material from the ward area. Unfortunately this alcohol consumption was often supplemented by stealing wine and brandy from the sick. Thefts from patients and bartering for medicines and food with them were less common in general hospitals, but quite commonplace in workhouse infirmaries.

This was where an unfortunate group, the pauper nurses, worked. They were women who had been admitted to the workhouse infirmaries when they were sick, on the understanding that when they were well enough they were to nurse the sick in return. Unpaid and having to nurse with little direct supervision from sisters of the quality coming through the Nightingale system, they were ill equipped to provide any meaningful care to the sick. Most of them were unable to read so there was always a difficulty for them in understanding medical instructions, even if they wanted to, let alone read prescriptions. Since physically able women absconded when they became well enough, only the old and weak were left to do this work. These poor souls were hardly able to lift a patient up the bed let alone provide basic care. Not surprisingly Florence Nightingale was not a devotee of the system that fostered pauper nurses, and was certainly not interested in training them. She maintained that she would not find among these women suitable candidates for an occupation which required, perhaps above every other occupation at that time, sobriety, honesty, trustworthiness, truthfulness, orderliness, cleanliness, good character, and good health. Her argument was that they had not shown honesty, not been trustwothy, or truthful, not been orderly or cleanly, not had good character or good health. She finally won the battle and introduced her new matrons and sisters into the workhouse infirmaries, so ending the tradition of pauper nursing.

But there were still other battles; she wrote on 29 May 1894 about one of the leading London hospitals:

The nurses . . . slept in wooden cages on the landing places outside the doors of the wards where it was impossible for any woman of character to sleep, where it was impossible for the night nurse taking her rest in the day to sleep at all owing to the noise, where there was not light or air.

However, there was now a matron in place making sure that 'a patient's arm did not linger too long on a nurse's waist'. Not only was she in charge of the nurses, she was also their moral guardian, setting standards of behaviour for her staff. This change in the moral approach to nurses was clearly in evidence by the end of the nineteenth century. At the Middlesex Hospital, London, the nurses wore dresses that had trains at the back so that when they bent over a bed their ankles would not be exposed to the view of the patients nor the male medical students. At this hospital the nurses were 'honoured' each day with a kiss from Miss Thorold, the Lady Superintendent.

Sisters were firmly in charge by the end of the nineteenth century and saw that the nurses carried out their instructions as well as the doctors'. Inevitably there were clashes between the older nursing sisters and matrons and the new ones. The new sisters were seen as too knowledgeable, interfering and bossy, and as threatening to the old guards' role. One notable example of this was at Guy's Hospital where Miss Burt was Matron. She had great difficulty introducing new clinical practices, let alone newly trained nurses, as many of the medical staff and sisters were quite happy with the system they were used to. She made it most apparent that she had no time for the nurses in post (the Betsy Prigs), who she felt spent much of their time in public houses and were unwilling to change. She thought they did little to relieve the suffering of the patients. To start with, she demanded that a uniform be worn by all the nurses and did not permit the wearing of jewellery. She instituted a system of rotating staff to different wards to develop their nursing experience. Her sisters were to take up her mantle and ensure that patient care was the foremost consideration.

So, with their increasing knowledge and confidence the sisters began to show their newly acquired competence. Many had developed to the point where they could now begin to help new housemen hone their own skills. Even so the new sisters were seen as a threat by some of the medical staff, who thought they might lose control over the patients' care. On the other hand there were many enlightened doctors who were only too pleased to place the day-to-day running of the wards in the capable hands of these ladies. The consultants were beginning to realize that they could more readily rely on the skills of these new, better-trained and more responsible sisters, and henceforward began to demand them to run the wards. Doctors began to take an increasing part in the appointment of these sisters. As the nineteenth century drew to a close, hospitals found that the quality and performance of nurses was improving under the supervision and tutoring of these highly trained sisters.

All this formed the basis for an evolution in the sister's role, incorporating rigorous nursing practice and an authoritarian ideology; this followed the prime Nightingale philosophy of centralizing power into her office. It worked, and through dedication and devotion the outstanding profession of nursing was born and from this point forward it was the ward sister who proved to be the backbone of the evolving health systems.

Another innovation for these sisters was the use of a communal dining-room for their main meal, which began to reduce the loneliness and isolation associated with their role. Years of guarding their authority had the effect of insulating them from the people who were their charges, the nurses. This loneliness was a factor for many generations of sisters. Norma Clacey (née Skehan) points out: 'As late as the 1950s we realized how institutionalized some of these sisters could be. Unmarried, most of them still lived in hospital.' When these ward sisters retired many had great difficulty adjusting to and managing the change to life outside nursing. Having lived in hospitals and hospital accommodation all their lives, shopping and budgeting were new experiences.

The Nightingale School trained almost two thousand nurses from 1860 to 1903. These nurses headed all major hospitals and wards in Britain and many of the hospitals abroad. Florence Nightingale's achievements were incredible in developing the skilled nursing profession that was essential to the progress of medicine. She sculpted the modern nurse out of material that at first was somewhat unpromising. From unprincipled and uneducated women without standards she introduced a disciplined, caring compassionate and educated force, with a qualified nurse leader at the head, the matron, and a leader of nursing at ward level, the sister.

3   The Martinets

They [sisters] did not as a rule mix socially or otherwise with those below them in the hierarchy. These sisters of long standing often looked with condescension on those who had only recently 'gone into blue'. In the wards they ruled with an iron hand.

G. Yeo, *Nursing at Bart's.*

'Being blued', 'going into blue' or 'being made up' were among the many expressions used when a nurse was promoted to sister. Promotion was based purely on merit; there were no rules other than a decision by the matron, sometimes in consultation with a doctor or the house committee. The decision could be given directly to a nurse in the matron's office, or even by a telephone call to the ward. No matter, it was a cause for great joy. From that moment onward she would be sister and would have her own ward and her own staff to mould to her standards.

At the turn of the nineteenth century these new ward sisters were expected to work from 8.00 a.m. to 10.00 p.m., with a three-hour break in the evening. Their salary was between £30 and £60 a year depending on the size and location of the hospital. Sisters were responsible for receiving and carrying out medical instructions and, in conjunction with the doctors, drawing up daily diet sheets. In addition, they were responsible for making daily rounds of the patients, for training probationers, and for reporting any changes to the matron. All new patients were received by the sister and allocated to their beds. They also served meals, conducted the medicine round, and supervised the entire organization of the ward.

The responsibility for the ward therfore rested with the sister as head nurse, with the nurses performing the clinical ward work and the helpers and maids performing the domestic duties. Each sister was provided with her own bedroom and in many hospitals a sitting room adjoining the ward, which meant that her whole day was spent in the ward environment. If she had any serious cases on the ward she could frequently be called out night after night. She received a salary, which was paid quarterly, but was not provided with any other rations except beer. She now worked more closely with the physician or surgeon to whose ward she was attached, and reported to the house surgeon in their absence any circumstances that called for immediate attention. She paid special attention to the severely ill cases on her ward. One surgeon reported of one sister: 'But for her unremitting care and womanly aid [the case] would not attain successful issue.' It was now expected that a sister would be the head nurse on all wards in all hospitals.

Advances in nursing practice were thus taking place, with the sisters accepting additional responsibility for the care of the sick. Sister posts more and more frequently were being filled by ordinary nurses, whose promotion was merited from length of service and presumed suitability. At the larger voluntary hospitals newly trained sisters were not expected to take charge of a ward immediately. Where previously many of them had been expected to the pick up their knowledge the best they could, they were now first taken on as supernumeraries. Unattached to a ward, they were placed in the matron's office, and by frequent errands to the wards they gained an insight into the duties they would undertake when they became attached sisters themselves. Following this probationary phase they were sent for short periods to work with a more experienced ward sister. Even then it was recognized that the probationary sister's nursing education was not complete; she had still much to learn which could only be obtained on the ward. The quality and speed with which she developed her skills were very much dependent on the assistance and guidance of the physician or surgeon to whom she was attached. What sort of ward sister she was to become depended a great deal on them.

With early nursing rooted firmly in the traditions of the military services and the religious orders, sisters in the post-Nightingale era were very strict in their approach to the nurses and the patients. Because of this, sisters have traditionally been unfairly stereotyped as embittered spinsters: martinets. They were in fact highly committed women determined that nursing was not going to revert to the lax standards and drunkenness of previous years. With a firm belief that 'discipline and hard work never hurt anyone', these sisters often seemed rather harsh on their junior nurses. The etiquette of hospital life was very rigid and non-observance certainly brought trouble. On the wards the nurses were instructed to stand in the presence of a sister and to address her respectfully at all times. Ward staff were only to be addressed as Sister, Nurse, or by their surname. To lean against a table or put her hands in her uniform pockets while the sister was speaking was seen as a sign of a want of natural politeness. It was further thought that a junior nurse who felt uncomfortable about rising when the sister approached her had a false pride unbefitting hospital work.

It should be pointed out, however, that it was not just in nursing that such rigid discipline applied. A history of a working life in a bank, shop, school or a newspaper office would all have similar tales of authoritarian management and subservience, and nursing was not the only profession in which a girl had to leave when she married or became pregnant.

Sisters were more than just attached to their wards: they were virtually married to their role. They were known only by the name of the ward – hence Sister Casualty, Sister Surgery or Sister Theatre, and at St Bartholomew's Hospital Sisters Faith, Hope and Charity in charge of the wards of those names. Other thought-provoking names were Cutting, Sweating and Diet. This practice was in many ways an ordination into the sisterhood of nursing in the same way that their nursing predecessors, the nuns, took on the name of a saint. It continued in many hospitals well into the middle of the twentieth century. Many sisters remained on their 'own' wards for the whole of their service, without a thought of moving on or advancing their careers further.

The first thing a new nurse learned was that Sister was in charge. If she did not quickly accept this she would soon land in trouble. Sisters could be gentle and nurturing or powerful and uncompromising. Their reputation ran ahead of them like a spectre, colouring the perceptions of new nurses before they set foot on the ward. Each one had her own idiosyncrasies and it was as well for a new nurse to get to know them beforehand, so that when ward allocation time came, she had some idea of what to expect. Almost all of them found that when they eventually worked with the sister, the spectre disappeared. The sisters then showed their warmer side and almost always acted with the patients' welfare at heart. Although nurses remember some who frightened them or who were bad managers, only rarely was their frightening reputation totally justified, and of course these sisters did not get the best out of their staff. The greatest respect of course went to the sister who was prepared to roll up her sleeves and join in the ward work.

Throughout the country ward sisters were becoming more respected in their own right, rather than because of the matron they worked for. They also became noted for their experience, devotion to work and diligence with the patients, gradually gaining respect within the hospitals. Physicians spoke of them having a fine commanding presence, a strict sense of discipline with their nurses, presence of mind and kindness of heart. The medical profession knew that without these better-trained sisters and skilled nurses the great advances in medical science would flounder.

For some young women in training, the uncompromising rigour of the daily routine did seem unduly strict. On entry to the ward, the sister would expect the following to be laid out like a kit inspection: instruments, rubber gloves, candles, ward silver, clean nit combs (all patients were regularly checked for nits), linen tea cloths, medicine cloths, hand towels, roller towels and bedpan covers. They were laid out in accordance with the sister's rules, the linen neatly folded with corners turned back. Finally, there had to be a full ink-well and clean nib for her pen. She counted the cutlery night and morning and if a single teaspoon was missing every locker and drawer was checked until it was found; moreover the nurses would not be let off duty until it was. Even the nursing staff were scrutinized. Hands, nails and aprons were inspected each morning and often before serving meals. Nurses did not usually object to this and thought it was a reasonable part of cleanliness in nursing.

This uncompromising discipline did get to one nurse, however. Vidie Lever, a student at St Thomas's Hospital explained: 'We would all stand when sister entered. She would say good morning everyone, but we were not expected to reply.' Sister would do her inspection of the nurses, take the hand-over and then do a full round of all the patients. The nurses would then sit at the table in the middle of the ward, where Sister allocated the work. 'I was terrified of her,' said Videy.

We had the clinic room at one end of the ward and the toilet at the other. You had these urine specimens and had to carry them up to the clinic room. I dropped them all in front of sister. It was no good saying, 'It was your fault, you make me so nervous.' But this dragon of a woman just said, 'Never mind nurse, I did that once.' I would do anything for her after that.

The sisters' rigorous approach extended to the annual ward and linen inventories, which were also conducted with military precision. No matter what was happening or what inconvenience they caused, they were carried out thoroughly, as in pre-National Health Service days everything had to be accounted for. Kay Riley found the whole thing quite amusing at St Thomas's Hospital, where each ward would be closed for a week for the inventory and spring cleaning.

There would have to be three spring dusters, three soft dusters and thirty thermometers, all laid out. It was like an army kit inspection with hot water bottles, bedpans, everything. It was quite comical really, if you did not have the sixty knives and forks you would charge to a ward upstairs and borrow whatever you were short of.

Linen inventory day was the same. Sister would be in early on that day and would direct the nurses to present all the linen, every item. The beds were made so that all the linen could be seen. Any linen not in use was openly displayed in alphabetical order on tables, even the dirty linen was counted. The most difficult part was ensuring that nothing was in the laundry on that day. Since institutional theft was not a major problem, with a little borrowing from other wards it was invariably a successful, if exhausting, day.

At the sister's right hand was the ward maid, who seemed to have as much authority as she did. The maid would work on the same ward for many years and knew the system better than anyone else, and woe betide a nurse who crossed her. But knowing the sister's singularities and the ward maid's foibles got a nurse out of many scrapes. If all were well, the maid would make the tea and would have various signals for nurses to 'escape' to the kitchen for a quick cup. But if anything had upset her they could forget such favours. It was therefore as well to get on the good side of these ladies, as it could stand the nurses in good stead for their time on the ward. The ward maids were so highly valued that many nurses thought they were probably more respected by the sisters than they were. Jenny Cooper remembers sitting a lady on a commode, screening her off, and looking with horror as a puddle of urine appeared on the floor, in her haste she had forgotten to place the bedpan under the patient. 'The maid flew into a fury and marched straight to Sister's office. Sister was certainly on the maid's side and harangued me in front of everyone.'

Jill Southern remembers:

> Our ward maid, my goodness she was a tartar. If she was in a mood, sometimes even Sister could not approach her. Upset her too early and she would be in a bad mood for the rest of the day. The way we got round this was to admire the polished floor and clean surfaces and let her see us tip-toe across her wet floor, she loved it.

Joan Baines worked on the children's ward at Manchester Royal Infirmary, where the cook was more in charge than the sister. If a nurse went into the kitchen she had to leave it in pristine condition, even the Aga cooker.

> No ward could keep the Aga clean, but she could, it was immaculate. She was fearsomely protective of her domain, there to cook all the children's meals, including the many diets required; she seemed to be in the unit the whole time. Throughout my career I found I could get on with anyone but I could never seem to get on the better side of her.

Autonomy within a ward was one thing but some nurses felt that it could be carried too far. One sister, for example, was very opposed to visitors. Said to be superb with the patients, she would make visiting time into an intimidating experience. Screens were placed across the entrance door to keep away interfering eyes and would only be removed at times to allow the flow of visitors to enter. A nurse recounted:

> After one hour, in which nurses would be set various tasks, the bell would ring. Sister would stand in the corridor outside her office with her arms folded in her uncompromising posture. When that bell was rung even relatives of the most gravely ill patients would be dismissed with little thought. She gave off an air that no one should talk to her and all visitors had to immediately vacate her ward.

Even for those days this seemed a callous abuse of power.

Many of the sisters Barbara Hare (née Clorley) remembered during her training in the early 1950s at Bolingbroke Hospital, Clapham Junction, had lost boyfriends and fiancés in the war. She felt they had therefore dedicated themselves to their role of nursing, and became sticklers for personal discipline. A task had to be finished even if it meant staying over an hour late. Knowing that they could be called back if they had not finished a job or if they had not put something away concentrated the nurses' minds. These sisters seemed to the students to be permanently in the hospital, and they were. Many still slept in a room attached to the ward. There they lived, ate and entertained, usually with other sisters, rarely with men. They also had pets, to which they naturally became very close. One sister was totally attached to her cat; when it died, she took it to the chapel and it lay there in its basket all night. Barbara Hare says:

> When we nurses had to go into the sisters' sitting rooms we stood straight, not quite to attention but it was done out of respect. Youngsters would scoff now but we all freely accepted the discipline, and were probably better for it. We did a 48-hour week, plus the extra hours you voluntarily or involuntarily put in. One of our last duties of the day was to count the laundry. I was ready to go off duty and went to Sister to excuse myself and was asked by her if I had counted the laundry. I replied no. She

sent me straight back to count it all before I could leave; I just accepted this, that was how it was.

Joan Page was training during the Second World War at the Queen's Hospital for Children.

One night I was woken by a loud bang and found my room covered in glass. A doodlebug had exploded next to the hospital. I hastily dressed, cap and all, and joined the other nurses in a walk in the dark across the yard to the basement of the hospital and up to the wards. All the children were unhurt, the cots having already been covered by mattresses, bent to form a protective arch over them. Once we had cleaned up and ensured all was well, we then went back to our rooms. On the way back I was met by the theatre sister and was shocked to see her wearing trousers instead of her uniform; we did not ever go anywhere without full uniform and to see a sister looking so casual was nearly as big a shock as the doodlebug. Back in bed, I was just about to fall asleep when the door opened and the matron and home sister walked in. 'Good gracious,' exclaimed Matron, 'Nurse Page must have slept through it all!'

Bathing facilities were the same for the sisters as for the patients and it was usually the junior nurse who had to clean and run her bath. It was highly important for sufficient screening to be provided so that the sister was not seen in her dressing gown. Many sisters who had trained at the turn of the century were very particular about their nightly bath. Joan Jenkins (née Horsley) explains her experience in 1932 at St George's Hospital, London. 'The wards were long with thirty-three beds and the sister's living room was off the centre of the ward, her room was delightful.' The night nurses were only invited into this room in the morning to give her the report. Joan was working on William King Ward and as junior nurse it was her job on a Friday night to disinfect the bath, screen the area off and then knock on Sister's door to say, 'Sister, your bath is ready.' Joan says:

Sister walked across to the bathroom in full uniform. On her return she came back in her dressing gown with a towel over her arm, she did not have her cap on. I said to Nurse Butt, 'Isn't it incredible, I have just seen sister without her cap.' It was incredible; I was astonished, and have never forgotten it. I then made sister a hot drink and took it to her room.

It was incredible; they would never allow themselves to be seen out of their uniforms, let alone partially dressed. They had to look immaculate at all times; their own standards were as important as the standards they so rigidly maintained on the wards. Inevitably, the rigid military style of discipline and the personal devotion to duty demanded could not be maintained in an evolving world. Gradually both came under pressure. Of course, not all sisters compromised willingly; some continued to maintain their formidable reputation and some continued to live in the sisters' home.

Doreen Tennant was on a ward sisters' course in 1954 and one of her placements was at Guy's Hospital, London.

Sister's sitting room was just off the ward and I was invited in to listen to the ward report and then stay for coffee. There was a door in the room and when I opened it there was a bed. I asked about the bed and she said it was hers. There was only a hand basin and no loo. I asked her where she went and she casually said, 'I have to use the ward or the corridor lavatory.'

The long tradition of prayer in hospitals continued up to the 1980s, and it was seen as important by both nurses and patients. Kay Riley was one of the last sisters to continue with ward prayers until her retirement in 1987. She would enter the ward, kneel down at the desk and say the following prayer:

Oh, Lord, our Heavenly Father,
Almighty and everlasting God,
Who hast safely brought us to the beginning of the day,
Defend us in the same with Thy mighty power,

And grant that this day we fall into no sin,
Neither run into any kind of danger,
But that all our doings may be ordered by Thy governance
To do always what is righteous within Thy sight.
Through Jesus Christ, our Lord, Amen.

She recalls:

In the east wing I had to use a microphone so the prayers could be transmitted to all bays. Hardly a day went by without the patients commenting on how helpful they were. The doctors also respected prayer time, and it did not matter what the religious denomination was, the patients respected it.

She also took some of the patients to the chapel service on Sunday, but this was her own decision and she would stay on an extra couple of hours to make up the time she had lost.

Times were changing, however, and not all sisters were comfortable with leading the prayers on the wards. Ruth Sanders, who also trained at St Thomas's Hospital, found that her lack of religious belief was often in conflict with those who were happy to continue this practice. When left in charge of a ward she continued the tradition but she would encourage one of the other staff to lead the prayers.

During her training at the London Hospital, Avril Vincent (née Williamson) was on her knees with the other nurses, the patients were in their beds and all were ready for the commencement of prayers. Sister solemnly entered, knelt on the hassock and started to read the London Hospital prayer, 'Almighty and Everloving God. . . .' Then she stopped and pointed. 'Who dusted under that bed this morning?' The dust seemingly had priority over God at that moment!

Clearly hospital life was strict and militaristic, but in a strange and sad way the system of nursing benefited from warfare. Two world wars killed millions of young men and altered the lives of millions more. It also damaged the marriage prospects of countless young women. War created a generation of spinsters from circumstances not choice, and it was from this group that the service gained the sisters who gave nursing respect and stability. They dedicated their lives to nursing, and with their selfless devotion they crystallized much that was good in nursing care.

4   Into the Lions' Den

You have been a staff nurse, you seem to have been a friend to
everybody, no more of that. There are going to be times when
you are going to have to put your foot down. You remember this,
if you get too friendly with anybody you cannot discipline them.

Advice to a newly promoted sister from a sister
at Leicester Royal Infirmary, 1953

The above advice was imparted by a respected senior colleague, but
similar words were said to another nurse and her colleagues by a
'dragon' of an assistant matron. At the nurses' prize-giving this lady
stood up and announced 'in her usual bossy manner': 'You remember this, girls, when it is time for you to be promoted to sister you
will find that you cannot be popular and have the respect of others
at the same time.' Unfortunately, she was neither popular nor
respected!

On the other hand the desire for popularity could backfire. During
training the nurses were allowed out from 7.30 to 10.00 p.m each
evening, and at ten o'clock sharp the home sister should have locked
the nurses' home door. But she did not have the necessary disciplin-
ary skills so the nurses could always string her along for at least
another ten minutes. Once the door was locked, assistance from a
boyfriend would see them into the grounds and hopefully into the
nurses' home through a window. This home sister also acted as sister
tutor, and she failed in this respect as well. A nurse reports:

It was a shame really. We had no respect for her; I suppose we
liked her but even to her face we were disrespectful, and she did

not have the skill or courage to do anything about it. It was a pity really, because she thought she was one of us, but it did not work.

Inevitably the proud day would come when a staff nurse would find herself promoted to the rank of sister, but nothing could prepare this new appointee for the first time she entered the sister's inner sanctum, their sitting or dining room. Jean Peach's first day as sister at the Royal Hospital, Sheffield, was unforgettable. She was for the very first time to enter the sisters' rest room.

So here was I about to enter the lions' den. How could I go about this, I thought. Some of these were the people I had been in fear of the whole of my training and I was about to join them. I foolishly knocked on the door, obviously announcing a new entrant, and walked in. A sea of blank faces and a deafening silence confronted me. In the few seconds it took me to get from the door to an empty seat I had been inspected from top to toe and many opinions had been formed. As I sat down their conversations began again, I no longer seemed to exist.

Daphne Fallows had the reassuring support of an experienced sister, Peggy Nuttall, for her first entrance into the sisters' lounge at St Thomas's Hospital. As she was hovering outside the door, not sure whether to enter or run away, it was Miss Nuttall who took her in. She just said, 'Come on, in we go,' and in they went. From that moment onwards she enjoyed the whole experience of being a sister and felt that she had been honoured in that promotion. She adds with a smile, 'Mind you it did help that I could then have my shoes cleaned as a privilege of being a ward sister.'

The telephonist knew about Norma Clacey's promotion to junior sister at the Royal Hospital, Portsmouth, before she did. Norma found the agony of walking into the sisters' sitting room made her legs wobble.

To walk into this room full of the sisters I had been so terrified of during my training, it was unbelievable. There they were, they had had their lunch and were having a cup of tea and talking about Christmas and the January sales. I thought, are these really the same sisters who gave me such a hard time as a student? One of them who I had been particularly wary of was so charming and actually asked me to teach her to knit.

Kay Riley's first appointment as a sister was as night assistant at St Thomas's Hospital, which gave her the dubious privilege of having her breakfast in the sisters' dining room. When she entered, the sisters were all sitting at their own tables. 'All I saw was *The Times* drop, revealing a row of faces. They all looked at me, they all looked at each other and then the papers shot up again.' Kay was not directed to a chair so sat at a table, only to be told that that was where Sister Charity sat. 'Do you know,' she said, 'I feel sure I could not have eaten my breakfast that morning, it was all such a blur.'

Entering the sisters' leisure area was undoubtedly daunting, but filling their shoes as relief ward sister was an unenviable position. Eager to have the opportunity to show off their own skills, the relief sister was not best positioned to carry change through. Vidie Lever felt she had a typically difficult time. The staff nurses often resented the relief sisters; after all they were there all the time and then along came someone who knew nothing about the patients. Moreover, the sister was intolerant of her system being changed.

> I naturally had to rely on the staff nurses for knowledge about patients. There was a round by the consultant, I had not had time to learn about the patients so had to take one of these resentful staff nurses with me. On another occasion I found nurses getting elderly patients out of bed without screening them, and doing their pressure areas.

She instructed the nurses to put screens round the beds and showed them how to do backs properly. The nurses in training were delighted; the trained nurses were not. When the permanent sister returned there was tremendous resentment from her also.

Moving from ward to ward could be equally difficult for student

50

nurses. Mary Hearn (née Brockway) had been working on a medical ward at Queen Alexandra Hospital, Cosham, and was eager to learn. The charge nurse had always answered her questions but said: 'I have enjoyed having you on the ward and I appreciate your enthusiasm and your desire to learn about nursing but a word of warning. I like this questioning, but many of the sisters of other wards may not.'

How right he was.

On the next ward the sister avoided answering any questions, but to be honest she was rare. Another of the sisters was very strict, she would give us hell for a week and then tell us how she had straightened you up. 'Now you are ready to work on my ward!' she would say, and to be fair we were.

Gwen Savage (née Brown), who initially trained at Kettering General Hospital, Northamptonshire, found her student years both rewarding and terrifying.

Rewarding when I felt I had done something right, praise was rare from a sister, and again rewarding when able to communicate with patients. Terrifying when I was on a ward where the sister was well known for being an ogre. Terrifying if I was a few minutes late, it did not matter about all the extra hours I had put in the day before. I still remember the feeling of guilt when asking Sister if I could go off duty.

Once on night duty Gwen burned her arm with an acid solution. There was no light in the sluice and she accidentally knocked a bottle out of the cupboard. Having to go to casualty for treatment, she was made to feel it was a great inconvenience for them and the night sister was furious, making it out to be her own fault. Health and safety was not quite the concern it is today.

Kay Riley had the misfortune to break the egg timer used for timing the sterilization of instruments. She immediately gathered the broken bits together in case someone else should be cut, cutting the top of her own finger in the process. This was reported to the sister, who accused her of not only being a fool, but of deliberately

doing it so that she could have time off sick. She was understand-
ably upset. At the end of her time on the ward the sister greatly
insulted her by suggesting that she would never make a nurse.
Fortunately the matron took a different view and sent her to a ward
with an extremely good sister. Kay went on to be a very successful
sister at St Thomas's Hospital. She also found that when promoted
to sister herself, the sister who had given her such a hard time
proved to be most thoughtful. Placed on night duty for the first
time, she had charge of the whole hospital. Now the Assistant
Matron, this sister wrote: 'Sister Riley, I do appreciate and understand how difficult it is on your first night and I want you to know
that you may contact me at any time if you have any problems at
all.'

She learned a great deal from these early experiences and when it
came to having her own ward she vowed to be more considerate to
both her patients and her staff.

> I tried to make work on my ward a fun experience, not flippant
> but fun. I used to arrange a pancake race on the ward every
> Pancake Day, and always ensured that there were drinks of
> sherry, champagne or Guiness before lunch on a Sunday. It was
> an attempt at making the ward as happy as I could. I also
> encouraged relatives to bring in the patients' pets.

Jean Holland and her colleagues were students at the
Manchester Royal Infirmary, where Matron Lucy Duff-Grant
explained to them: 'There will be times when you will be blamed
for things you weren't responsible for, so I do not want you nurses
running to me for every little infraction.' These wise words were
not enough for Jean on one occasion. Most of the sisters were kind
and considerate – some were described as 'sweethearts' – but two
were not, and one of these was working in the out-patient department. In her senior year, Jean was working in the septic hand clinic
with a young doctor. 'This battle-axe raged in, asking why we had
such a long line of patients waiting. I explained that we were working as fast as we could and that the load was very heavy.' The sister
stormed, 'If you and Dr D— didn't fraternize so much you would
get more done'. Forgetting matron's words for a moment she

replied, 'You are wrong, and I am quitting!' When the opportunity offered itself she went to see matron to offer her resignation. Matron pointed out that insubordination was not tolerated and told her to go to her room and report to her the next day. She did. Matron asked if she still wanted to leave, Jean said no and was sent back to work in out-patients. Sister very gently welcomed her back and placed her back in the septic hand clinic.

When Ruth Sanders began her training at St Thomas's Hospital in the 1970s, many sisters still seemed unapproachable; they looked very superior in their blue uniforms, with special hats with strings tied under the chin. One of them was so regal in her bearing that she thought of her as the Queen; majestically she would always walk just slightly behind everyone else.

You automatically felt she was above the rest of us, a very scary figure, a person you just knew you would never get close to. But my goodness she knew us students; she seemed to know so much about us. One way or another she sussed us all out. When this sister was on duty the patient always came first, noticeably first. She would not be in the office like some other sisters, she would be active round the beds.

To relieve the tension of work the nurses would have moments of fun. Working at St Nicholas Hospital, Plumstead, Audrey Jones (née Cole) found that the sisters in her day were like gods. If they had the slightest fault or odd habit, therefore, the students would mimic them. On one ward was a sister whom they called 'Haggis' because she had trained at the Edinburgh Royal Infirmary. A very straight-backed, stern-looking woman, it seemed she was omnipotent. She had a habit of appearing on the ward at any time, day or night. Audrey and a colleague were relaxing in front of the ward kitchen fire after they had prepared all the trays ready for next morning's break-fast. Her friend was having a cigarette, the sin of all sins. She puffed away, saying, 'All we need is bloody old Haggis to come now and I would be for it.' Old Haggis had quietly entered the kitchen and was standing on the opposite side. 'I could not say anything to my friend, nor did old Haggis. She just quietly turned and left, knowing that she did not have to say anything. Looking back now, old Haggis was probably in her late thirties!'

Joan Eddings (née Bains) commenced training at the Westminster Hospital in 1940. For the first two years the nurses lived in the hospital at Hyde Park Corner. At Lyons Corner House they could buy a brunch for 1s 3d (6p) and for an extra 9d (4p) a rainbow ice cream would be added. This treat would be accompanied by the music of Geraldo and his Orchestra. At the Westminster Hospital the theatre sister, who was affectionately known as the 'White Cat', was a popular, tall, imposing blond who treated the new nurses who worked in theatre very kindly. The night sister was less affectionately known as the 'Black Cat'. It was her ability (as with many night sisters) to enter the wards quietly, often catching the nurses off guard. But as Joan pointed out:

> This was unfair really as she was most helpful to us as junior nurses, understanding how difficult it was for us on night duty. Mind you she did keep us on our toes. When we knew she was on the way we would certainly jump to it, and if there was a medical student having a cup of tea, off he would be sent.

For Wendy Wild one sister at the Royal Free Hospital, London, was the most terrifying sister one could ever work for. She had tightly curled red hair and a brusque manner. Wendy had the misfortune to be sent to the ward, where she felt she did quite well at keeping out of Sister's way, but that did not last. There were mackintosh sheets on the beds and the nurses used to wash them and hang them out of the window to dry.

> I don't suppose I should have, but I hung a couple out and one fell into the yard three floors down. I had hardly got out of the sluice before I heard, 'Where is that student throwing things out of my window.?' Somehow in that short time someone had phoned sister from a lower-floor ward.

Later this sister nearly ended Wendy's career. She describes herself then as a fairly timid character but one day she took a deep breath, approached the sister and said that she felt she was not learning very much. The sister more or less told her to get on with it. Wendy said, 'One morning I could not face going in; instead I got myself ready and went home. I walked over a mile to the station, then had a long train journey. By the time I got home I had not regretted it, my parents had already been told and were expecting me.' She was allowed by the matron to take two weeks' leave with her parents to recover and then went back to complete her training, but she did not go back to that ward. Wendy can now look back on this experience and recognize the importance of the sister as head of a team of nurses.

Pip Bradstock (née Roberts), who trained at Cheltenham School of Nursing, found that the worst sisters she encountered were those who shouted at staff in the open ward. Strict sisters she did not mind, but those who shouted at staff in front of patients she could not accept. Though they were rare, new students would find this difficult to take and Pip spent a lot of her time supporting them. On the other hand she added, 'You always recall with affection the sisters who taught you, even if it was a hard lesson sometimes!'

When she was a student nurse Sylvia Kemp overslept and consequently a call came from the sister in the theatre department to tell her to get out of bed, get dressed and get to theatre. She very kindly added that she should have her breakfast before she went.

I thought, isn't she lovely? Sister nodded when I got to theatre and did not refer to my lateness. At four in the afternoon it was time for the late-duty staff to go to tea. She delegated the staff and included me. I replied, not me I am due off duty at five. 'Oh no you are not young lady,' said Sister, 'You are here till seven-thirty.'

Mary Hearn can still never smell Elizabeth Arden's Blue Grass perfume without shuddering. The nurses could smell the perfume coming long before a particular sister entered the ward. On the ward she had two tropical fish tanks; if the fish were all right, then so was sister. If one of the fish was not looking too good, she would busy herself changing the water, turning the oxygen up and generally fiddling about. If one died she would be a tyrant for the day. 'I have to admit that once or twice we nurses removed a fish that was not looking too healthy because sister would be so horrible. Amazingly she never noticed!'

Trained at the Royal Masonic Hospital, London, Liz Carter (née Ebdon) was on night duty for the first time. Following a quiet night she and her colleague proceeded to make all thirty beds to help the day shift. Very pleased with themselves they handed over to the day nurses, who were delighted. While they were having their well-earned breakfast in the dining room they were interrupted by a nurse who told them Sister wanted to see them immediately. Not quite sure why, they returned to the ward to find the sister standing with her arms folded by a bed. She pointed out that they had put a sheet on upside down and the hospital emblem was not showing. 'I am not accepting this shoddy work; as I do not know how many more beds are incorrectly made, you can strip them all and make them again!'

Sue Clemments was a third-year student at Great Ormond Street Hospital for Sick Children, London, when she was left in charge of a ward one evening. She was going towards the sluice room when a large area of water confronted her. The junior student had left the sterilizer running. Anxious at what the sister would say to the student, she grabbed the dirty linen skip and some clean sheets and started to dam the water. Sister came back from supper and said, 'I did not expect the floor to be cleaned at this time in the evening nurse but while it is wet we had better get on with it.' With that she set about cleaning the place up and never said a word to the student when she came back.

When Pauline Ellison (née Lawrence) commenced her general nurse training at St Thomas's Hospital she expected to meet a more autocratic type of sister than those she had worked with during her psychiatric training at St James Hospital, Portsmouth. However, although there were strict hierarchies, there were no autocrats. The sisters were younger than she expected, and their styles of management different. 'Trained by the more traditional sisters, they were undoubtedly brought up in the proper style of Nightingale training, which was to train others.' She felt the sisters were taught to pass learning on for others to deliver the best care, and that teaching was part of that process. Knowledge was clearly not exclusive; it was there to share.

The most dedicated sister Joan Chambers met was at the Firvale

Infirmary, Sheffield. The patients were mostly elderly, many from its workhouse days. Sister Walker was totally committed to their care; she was what would now be called a workaholic. She seemed to Joan to be on the ward the whole time, dashing here and there, and always available when a problem arose. Keeping up with her was a breath-taking experience. She chatted and joked her way through any situation but she was also a strict disciplinarian, so there was never any danger of a nurse taking advantage of her good nature. She led by example, sometimes doing duties a junior was expected to do, and as a consequence was greatly respected. 'She was brilliant,' Joan remembers, 'but she nearly spoiled it for me on my following wards. I did not meet another sister who came up to her standard.'

Consultants could appear extremely remote to junior nurses, but it was recognized that many sisters and consultants had a special relationship that transcended the usual stuffiness between doctors and nurses at one time. They understood each other, respected each other's area of expertise and tolerated each other's singularities. Margaret Webster pointed out that as ward sister she had to keep a close eye on all aspects of the ward, irrespective of the speciality. She often had to guide both junior and senior doctors if they were uncertain; 'We sort of took them under our wing until they gained more confidence.' She added, 'We worked together, but I was the boss.' As a young medical student at University College Hospital, Dr Ray Radford grew to respect ward sisters but in particular the sister in charge of the diabetic ward.

She was highly knowledgeable. She was renowned throughout the medical school. The consultants had enormous respect for her and she would get many of us medical students out of trouble if we miscalculated the medication or wrongly diagnosed the illness. Usually she managed to give us this advice just in time for the consultant's round.

Extremely formidable in their approach to the nurses, these same sisters could nevertheless have their moments of romance. When she was appointed a staff nurse in the ear, nose and throat department, Margaret Ollerton (née Woodington) worked for a sister at Manchester Royal Hospital who was very strict with the nurses but quite openly having a relationship with an older anaesthetist.

Everybody knew, it was the talk of the department. They would disappear into the surgeon's room and lock the door. Nobody seemed to mind it; it was so lovely for them. They would also dine out at a local restaurant. This was of course in the days when it was still not acceptable for medical staff and nurses to be in any sort of relationship let alone a close one.

Jean Garner observed a similar situation. She was so in awe of the sisters that it came as quite a shock to realize that they were ordinary people with ordinary feelings. Trained at the Royal Hospital, Sheffield, towards the end of the Second World War, she commented:

I was a very unworldly eighteen-year-old. Sister Grant was someone I both feared and revered, almost like a mother. Imagine my surprise when I saw her out with a man that I thought I recognized. There was no doubt the next time I saw them together, they were in the doorway to the sisters' home and he was kissing her; then I recognized him, he was a hospital engineer. It was like finding my mother with another man; I could hardly look her in the eye. It seems so silly now but it certainly was not then.

Although the standards of work on the wards were never allowed to lapse, now and again the regime of harsh discipline could be relaxed, particularly at Christmas. Few sisters would allow themselves the frivolity of tinsel in their hair, but they would make similar concessions for their nurses. All nurses were expected to be on duty over the Christmas period and it was a time that everyone looked forward to for many weeks. Unlike today, it was well into December before Christmas decorations appeared in the shops and they were very often not put up in homes and on hospital wards before Christmas Eve.

Carol singing around the hospital was a special event not to be missed; it was both meaningful and poignant. Whether they were believers or not, the staff would join in with great gusto. The starting point was usually the main hall where they would all congregate on the staircase; here the singing was said to be at its best. All the staff wore full uniform. The nurses would turn their capes so that the red side was outwards, and each would carry a candle. There would then be a crocodile procession of staff through the corridors and into the wards, led by the matron. The ward lights would be dimmed. 'Can you imagine it,' said Joan Eddings; 'the stillness on the wards, the sound of the choir in the corridor getting slowly louder and then the candle-lit procession entering the darkened ward?' It was such a powerful, emotional, magical experience that no one involved would ever forget it.

On the maternity wards both the nursing staff and the mothers would join in. Mothers who could sit in a chair would take their babies from the cots and line the corridor to listen to the carollers as they passed. The first Christmas baby was always a special celebration. A cot was ornately decorated in tinsel and baubles and great delight was taken in placing the new 'Christmas Day' baby there. There was always great interest from the local newspaper in this wonderful event.

Throughout the country, nurses celebrated Christmas with early morning visits to hospital chapels. For the patients, services were held on the wards and communion could be taken. Patients stayed in hospital for much longer and nurses worked long hours, so they really got to know their patients. 'Our sister,' said Jane Prichard, who trained at Doncaster Royal Infirmary, 'was marvellous, as big in heart as anyone could be. She organized ward concerts and singsongs the year round, but Christmas was always her forte. Never to be left out she would sing in her strong Yorkshire accent any carol the patients requested.'

Liz Carter always remembers Christmas as an outstanding experience. Each ward at the Royal Masonic Hospital had a separate theme: Christmas across the world, a traditional Christmas, or a colour theme such as red, silver and blue. The nurses would go to Covent Garden to collect any decorations that could be spared. 'On the morning before Christmas Eve,' Liz remembers, 'we would go in full uniform and collect all the Christmas trees, holly, mistletoe, fruit, in fact anything they had left. The vendors were wonderful to us.' So Christmas would be a time of transformation on the wards. With no strict fire regulations, decorations were everywhere: there was holly round the windows, mistletoe over the doors, paper decorations festooning the walls and paper chains pasted together by patients and staff hung from light fitting to light fitting. Sometimes certain unsavoury items, best not mentioned, would be suspended from various vantage points. These would be a great source of amusement; a lecture by sister on keeping decorum was in the main ignored! Father Christmas came to visit the ward on Christmas morning with a sack full of presents for the patients and usually also for the staff; patients invariably guessed who was in the costume. Off-duty staff would find the energy to get to the lunchtime celebrations, where the consultant traditionally sliced the turkey. It never ceased to amaze nurses how Sister could be so different on this day from the rest of the year.

The nursing staff would have spent evenings wrapping presents they had bought throughout the year. David Beach, who worked at the Manor Hospital, Walsall, in 1962, remembers selling cups of tea to visitors and raffles on the ward to earn the money for the celebrations and presents. 'If we did well, every patient and nurse on the ward got a present.' In the morning carols were sung and the children would be dressed in party frocks, which were kept from year to year, for just this occasion. Sue Carter remembered that at Great Ormond Street all the children who were able would be taken to the main party. It was enormous work for the nurses, but tremendously worthwhile. Here patients got presents, crackers, funny hats and plenty of food. Anyone wanting to fund-raise for hospitals invariably chose children's wards. The Royal Yacht personnel adopted one in Portsmouth every Christmas. The sailors would bring a cake that had been made while the ship was at sea. It was a big day for the nurses and a big day for the sailors. One year one of the children nearly let the nurses down with his honesty. A senior officer came to the ward smelling a little the worse for drink; when he got too close to this particular boy he called out, 'Phew, you don't half smell of beer, mister.'

Towards the end of the Second World War Joan Page remembers the American Eagle Squadron visiting Queen's Hospital for Children with toys. All the children, with the exception of the very young or the very ill, went on foot or in chairs, cots or beds to the out-patients' hall. There they were entertained, and an airman dressed as Father

Christmas gave each child a toy.

I remember one boy who was on the ward because he had otitis media but was also very withdrawn. He backed away from the airman, who was offering a toy gun. With encouragement from us he grabbed it and tucked it under his arm and there it remained. I had to explain that the boy was autistic, but we knew very little about this handicap at that time.

The fancy dress party for staff at Christmas would allow nurses to be very innovative. The staff of the neurosurgery ward at the Royal Hospital, Sheffield, where Margaret Webster was sister, went dressed up as nuts and crackers. The nurses put eight staff in a bed, top to toe, dressed as a bunch of crackers. The only problem was the weight; on their journey around the hospital one of the bed wheels punctured the floor in the main hall, pitching them all on the floor! Matron had to reprimand them, but she obviously had a job keeping a straight face.

Official Christmas parties on the other hand could be an ordeal. When Beryl Varilone was in nurse training at Devizes and District General Hospital they were given the privilege of having a Christmas party at the nurses' home with Matron officiating. It was held in the sitting room, which was not very big. Matron sat there watching and listening to everything. The nurses had to file past and present their boyfriends. This caused great anxiety, as each nurse looked for a sign of disapproval in Matron's eye if the boyfriend was not up to standard. They were then expected to move around the room socializing, with a plate of food in one hand and a drink of lemonade in the other. A gramophone would be playing but none had the nerve to dance. At ten o'clock sharp, Matron would rise, heralding the end of the evening's festivities. Boyfriends were immediately seen off – no late passes that night.

On the wards the medical students would invariably attempt to kiss the sisters. The sterner the sister, the greater the challenge; of course they would have a handy piece of mistletoe in their pockets. The very brave would try to kiss the matron and the home sister, with varying degrees of success. The consultants and their families and the Lord Mayor would visit the wards, and of course they were treated with due respect and dignity.

There were also Christmas dinners for the staff, and a pantomime or resident show. These were opportunities for a hilarious romp. Put on by a small group of dedicated staff the costumes were made by the nurses, using the most colourful of materials; they were described as works of art. The shows were often a chance to lampoon the senior medical and nursing staff, who would sometimes join in the shows.

Matron's ball would mark the end of the Christmas and New Year festivities. A more formal occasion, this was seen as a gift from Matron to all the staff of the hospital. A time of unique family atmosphere, it was a time when junior staff realized that they belonged to more than just a hospital.

When Christmas was over, sisters would revert to their old selves. Training at the Princess Alice Hospital, Eastbourne, in 1942, Edith Chaplen and a friend, being rather young, constantly received the attentions of the many young men there; the hospital was full of wounded servicemen. Following Boxing Day they were left in charge of the ward while the sister went for her tea break. They were very busy, but those soldiers who were able to walk decided to continue the fun. They bundled the nurses into an empty bed and threatened them with many dire consequences, including getting their own back with an enema, 'like the one you gave us last week nurse!' Horror of horrors, just at that very moment the sister returned, accompanied by the matron. She was not the sort of sister to accept such behaviour at any time, but especially in front of the matron, and they expected to be suspended at the very least. Fortunately they were simply warned that any future such behaviour would mean instant dismissal. The soldiers were extremely sorry for the trouble they had caused and could not do enough for them to make up.

It was the same for Margaret Webster. One of her Monday jobs was to wash the light shades, and to do this she had to stand on a chair. The ward overlooked the matron's office and she was seen by the administration sister 'having a bit of fun' with a young dental student, a patient with osteomyelitis. This sister was a dragon of a woman, to be avoided at all costs. She immediately charged up to the ward and spoke to Margaret's sister. Margaret was told off in no uncertain terms. 'My punishment from sister was to give the young man an enema.' Presumably looking at the young man from this vantage point was designed to cool any ardour.

There have been as many different sisters as there are individual personalities. They stamped their own character on nursing and on their wards. In the following chapters we will see how they stamped their identity on each speciality.

5   Matron's Lieutenants

> Striding purposefully towards us her elbows pumping the air she
> had a string of nurses in her trail. She looked to me for all the
> world like a mother hen with her chicks.
>
> Monica Mattison's first sight of a home sister
> at Scarborough General Hospital, 1943

When Florence Nightingale began her plans to open the nursing
school at St Thomas's Hospital she had already decided that the
probationers should reside in a suitable home in the grounds of the
hospital. Her intention was that it should have a 'real' homely atmosphere. The original site was at Southwark; it was an imposing building, specifically given over to this use. When a new pupil arrived,
usually by horse and trap, Mrs Wardroper, the matron, or one of the
sisters welcomed them. When a new location at Lambeth was made
available the pupils were transferred there. Here, the home sister
would greet them.

Until the late 1960s hospitals were run centrally, with the matron,
the hospital secretary and a medical officer administering them.
Assistant matrons and administration sisters supported this central
organization by running a number of departments. Various roles were
included under this grouping, including Home Sister, Sister
Housekeeping, Sister Linen Room, Sister Holidays and Sister of the
Ward Maids. Often older sisters, they were also the keepers of hospital traditions and the maintainers of standards among the nurses.

At St Thomas's Hospital, Mrs Wardroper oversaw the training
school and the nurses' home as well as the hospital, but it soon
became apparent that the combined demands were too much. The

hospital committee decided to appoint someone who could assist her by taking charge of the nurses' residence. This assistance initially came from Miss Torrance, who quickly became known as Home Sister. She was not long in the post when she left to marry, and was replaced by Miss Machin, who in turn was succeeded by Miss Crossland. Miss Crossland had first come to St Thomas's as a probationer in 1874. Never a ward sister herself, she had previously been a governess, and this seems to have stood her in good stead. Her contribution to the welfare of the nurses and their training cannot be too highly praised. Undoubtedly devoted to her work, her post as Home Sister proved to be a model for other hospitals to follow. After an initial settling-in period, Mrs Wardroper wrote to Miss Nightingale, 'I know it will give you pleasure to hear that Miss Crossland makes a capital sister of the nurses home.'

The post of Home Sister was never going to be easy. Miss Nightingale thought that it would be the most trying and responsible position in the hospital, almost more so than that of Matron, 'because the home sister's charges changed continually'. Few are the perfect matrons, she would caution, but fewer still are the perfect home sisters. More than one probationer's father looked on the home sister as if she were something of a replacement mother. It may well be that at the end of the nineteenth century she was more likely to have been a replacement nanny or upper housemaid, as many of the applicants were ladies from higher-class homes and were used to having these people in their lives.

Living in the nurses' home was compulsory for the probationers. However, not all wanted to enjoy the dubious pleasures of living in that restrictive world. Pleading in the *Nursing Times* in 1908 for a system of living out as well as living in, Lucy Ashby was confronted by strong encouragement on the one hand and stiff resistance on the other. She replied to one objector, Miss Hobbs, Secretary of the Royal British Nurses' Association, and one of the nursing profession's most able leaders, who had expressed a fear that living out would lead to impaired digestion, owing to the hurried meals that would result. Lucy Ashby wrote that it was well known that meals in most hospitals were about as hurried as they could be. Half an hour was allowed for each meal, but it often happened of course, that a nurse's duties prevented her from getting down at the proper time, with the result that she was very hurried. She argued that the nurse had to finish her meal at the prescribed time, no matter when she had begun. She continued, 'Does not Miss Hobbs agree that living out would tend rather to improve things in this direction? Would not a walk from home or lodgings to hospital after a hurried meal be less harmful than the immediate beginning or return to work as at present?' The result of the living in system she felt was that nursing was being deprived of hundreds and potentially thousands of women who were no doubt particularly well fitted for the work.

Nurses were used to a considerably more restricted life at the end of the nineteenth century than today. The restrictions and discipline were highly acceptable to their parents, who felt it was essential for the safety and moral welfare of their daughters. Up to the Second World War it was a rather cloistered life, with great emphasis on the moral and religious welfare of the nurses; attendance at church was normally compulsory. The dining room usually contained long tables, and speaking was not allowed until grace was said. The home sister served the lunch and maids brought it round. The home sister kept a strict and watchful eye on her charges; one nurse was seen putting salt on another nurse's pudding for a joke, and without further ado, the home sister ensured that the offender ate it.

Monica Mattison (née Johnson), who trained at Scarborough General Hospital during the Second World War, remembers the home sister charging across the grounds, with her and the other nurses valiantly trying to keep up. Flinging open the main doors she would usher her nurses in and off she would go again down the corridors, detailing nurses off here and there. She was described as a wonderful lady, and ensured that there were always flowers from the garden for the young nurses to take home. If there were any extra rations left, she knew which nurse's family would most benefit. The normal wartime weekly ration was 2 ounces of butter, 4 ounces of sugar, 2 ounces of cheese, 2 rashers of bacon and 2 eggs. When the nurses had a sleeping out pass they went to the housekeeper sister who gave them their day's ration.

Discipline started on the first morning. The home sister would say, 'Now girls, change into uniform and let me see how you look.' Then she would point out any infringement of dress, particularly make-up, jewellery, watches and hats. Hats and studs were the bane of a new nurse's life, and the most heinous of crimes was to have hair dangling beneath one's hat. Folding, pinning and pleating the cap, and securing it to the head, was a work of art, achieved with a wide assortment of pins. The nurse was not allowed to leave the nurses' home without being checked from head to foot. The apron had to be exactly the same length as the wearer's dress and precisely 8 inches from the floor. Every sleeve puff had to droop at the same angle and each cap had to fit snugly round the compulsory head-bun.

The home sister also ensured that lights were out on time, and that permission for late passes had been sought from the matron's office. No musical instruments or animals were allowed in rooms, and certainly no men. She inspected the rooms and ensured that they were clean and tidy. The nurses were only allowed seven or eight items on their dressing tables so that it was easy for the maid to do her work, and were not allowed to leave clothes in the bathroom for the same reason. She also acted as policeman. When Lesley Smith commenced her nurse training in 1936 at the Herrison Hospital, Dorchester, she had what little money she possessed stolen from her room. She reported this to the home sister, who immediately informed the matron. They investigated, but discovered nothing, so told her to be more careful and that was the end of it.

When nurses were unfortunate enough to be in sick bay or having problems, the home sister would come into her own. Vidie Lever, a St Thomas's Hospital nurse, explained:

> One evening I was crying on my bed when Home Sister came in. She asked what was the matter. I explained that my mother was ill with cancer. She was on a gynaecology ward. Home Sister said, 'Don't you worry, we will see Matron in the morning.' She came with me to see Matron and while I was there, Matron not only arranged for a consultant to visit my mother, she also arranged for me to be sent home in a taxi. Some months later my mother was dying with terminal cancer and I was allowed leave from my training to look after her. Those two ladies showed real compassion to me.

The home sister was not only in charge of the nurses' living conditions she was also responsible for their moral welfare. Dr George

Steele was wooing his future wife at Manchester Royal Infirmary in the late 1940s and, as with any young man, the home sister made it difficult. George was a medical student but this was no advantage; in fact he was probably treated with more suspicion. Like a potential mother-in-law, the home sister would put obstacles in the way of wooing, even for those staff nurses and sisters who lived in the home. Joan, the subject of his attentions, went from student nurse to sister but the restrictions changed little. The facilities for visits in the nurses' home were most forbidding, with male visitors only allowed through the door with express prior permission. The home sister observed all contact from her office, which was situated directly opposite the visitors' room. With considerable ingenuity the door to the visitors' room had been modified so that it could not be shut; the hinges had been adjusted so that it swung permanently open. There were only two chairs, 'sparser than the interview room in a police station,' George remembers. One can see why the name for many nurses' homes became 'Virgins' Retreat'.

These facilities had not changed one bit when Joan was a ward sister and George was on his first leave from the army. Although they were newly married, it was pointed out that a nursing sister 'living in' was to be available for hospital duties at all times – there was certainly no consideration for compassionate leave in those days. The only alternative was a room at the Essex Hotel, a run-down building across the road from the Infirmary. At night it was illuminated with a neon sign, but the tubes for the E and the S were unlit (or removed), so the sign read '– – SEX HOTEL'. George and Joan caused some interest when registering; being genuinely married, they registered under their true name of Mr and Mrs Steele.

Nurses did not always want to be kept on such a strict rein, but the home or night sister would diligently do their round in the evening and expect nurses to be in their rooms on time. This could be diffi-cult, as many nurses left the wards only half an hour before lights out, if they were lucky, but the lights would be switched off regardless. Those nurses having a night out also had to be in on time. At one hospital a nurse was caught coming through the french windows that she had previously left open and was apprehended by the home sister. It was not her first time, and she was told to go to her room and not to report for duty next morning, but be in uniform. She was taken to the matron's office, where she was told to pack her bags, place her uniform on the bed and leave at once. Her colleagues did not see her again.

Margaret Morris (née Window) and some friends at the Miller Voluntary Hospital, Greenwich, came in late one evening and found the home sister sitting in the dark waiting for them. Expecting the worst they explained that they had been out to an old-time dance evening. The home sister wanted to know more, and they explained that they had danced the lancers, the valetta, the gavotte and other dances. Highly interested she became so caught up in her own reminiscences that she forgot about their lateness. She also ignored the food they had brought in, not too cunningly concealed beneath their coats.

Marion Dyson (née Upson) lived in the nurses' home at Huddersfield Royal Infirmary. Her friend Madge Bracken was somewhat unfortunate in having to share her room with a girl who was in the Salvation Army. Regardless of any restrictions, as a member of the band she had to practise on her instrument. She played the cornet and would drive Madge mad, as well as the other nurses near the room; she did more practice on the cornet than she ever did on her nursing subjects.

Living in the nurses home was bad enough; it was even more hazardous if one lived in the same home as the matron. Sylvia Kemp's room was above the ground-floor flat of Miss De La Court, Matron of Queen Alexandra Hospital, Cosham. One day Miss De La Court did a ward round and Sylvia was the only nurse free to escort her.

> I took some flack on that round I can tell you. An hour later I was going off duty and there was Matron in her garden. I had to pass her but wanted to ignore her because she had given me such grief. I tried to slip round the back without her seeing me, but a voice boomed, 'The front door is open, Sylvia.' I ignored her. 'The front door is open dear.' I could not dare ignore her again so I went in with just a slight slam of the door.

Jacqueline Collett caught the tail end of living in when she trained at the same hospital in the 1960s. Part of the nurses' home was adapted for the use of student nurses; the rest was the sister's home.

'It was no less strict,' she said. 'All the sisters were still single at this time. It was they who had the grand staircase and carpets in their part of the house and the student nurses who had a grotty staircase and lino at the rear of the house.' The sisters ate in a separate dining area. At this time the students did not resent it because they felt that the sisters had earned this privilege. 'I know the modern nurse would not understand this and would resent even the thought of it but they had earned their position. We did not moan, nobody bewailed this, it was OK. We felt safe on our bit of lino and had fun with saying, "I dare you to walk on that bit of carpet." '

Even sisters had to earn their privileges sometimes. Margaret Webster at Queen Elizabeth Hospital, Birmingham, recalls, 'I was not allowed a front-door key to the nurse's home until I had been a sister for three years.' Later, as a sister tutor in 1955 she refused to continue the practice of supervising student nurses cleaning their rooms in the nurses' home, and the matron readily accepted this. Being observed or inspected had been a routine part of a new nurse's activity for the first three months of their training.

For Kate Fisher at the South Yorkshire Asylum in the 1930s, living in meant living in the side wards of the asylum, off the main patients' wards. Mainly she thought they were there for the benefit of the night sisters, who would call them out if the night staff were having difficulty with a patient. At meal times they would go to the nurses' mess room and help themselves to the food. If they were late the food would be gone. After many complaints a sister was appointed by the matron to see that food was distributed properly. For tea they would have bread and butter; half of the week they would have marmalade, the other half honey, and once a week celebration cake. She felt she would have done better at the Bristol General Hospital – the nurses had been having jam every day and cake three times a week since 1920.

In the nurses' home at St Nicholas Hospital, Plumstead, was a 'wonderful' housekeeping sister who used to like a drop of gin. Audrey Jones and some friends were on night duty during rationing. 'Being young girls, we were constantly hungry, so we approached sister and explained this to her. Sister said, "Come on kids", and slightly wobbly she proceeded to take us to the kitchen.' They always knew when she had had a drink; she would smile sweetly and call them kids. She opened the pantry door and then went off without explanation, leaving them there. 'Well you can imagine it; we stuffed food in our clothes even our knickers while we could. When she came back I was on a ladder, bulging with food. I am sure she was too tipsy to know, and off we scuttled.'

Joan Page was appointed Home Sister and administrative relief at the Guy's Hospital unit at Orpington in 1954. This was a hutted establishment and nurses would change over in groups of about twenty. On change-over days Joan had to count out the soiled bed linen, clean the rooms and make the beds ready to welcome the new girls coming in. She organized teams of cleaners to work with her as they went from hut to hut. 'The assistant home sister normally helped me but on one occasion, All Saints' Day, she had gone to mass. I was not amused.' One night the phone by her bedside rang, but no one spoke. 'It was twilight, so I hastened up the hill to the nurses' accommodation and found that a nurse had phoned me. She had woken to find a man standing by her bed looking at her; he fled when she woke. The nurse was terrified.' Joan advised all the nurses to ensure that their doors and windows were locked. The man continued to prowl the area, but despite frequent visits from the police and night patrols by Joan he evaded capture. One evening Joan actually caught sight of him. She gave chase but he disappeared in an old part of the building. Joan was convinced that he must know where to hide. He did; when he was eventually caught they found he was a member of the hospital staff.

For many decades the home sister undoubtedly took a great load off the matron's daily work schedule but she was not the only sister to do this. As head of the nursing department, matron could not be everywhere. She had her own administration department of deputy matron, assistant matron and administration sisters, who were her eyes and ears in the various nursing sectors. This administration team did everything from clinical issues for patients to providing nursing and domestic staff cover, organizing training and ensuring cleanliness and order. Between them they were the orchestrators of the nursing administration system and also a team of quality controllers before quality control was thought of. The system worked well at that time, but it will not be seen in our hospitals again.

Sister Laundry and Sister Linen were highly important people in the smooth running of the hospital, managing the laundry girls and the linen store. The laundry prided itself on turning out the cleanest and best laundered items. The main linen store was virtually out of bounds to nurses, only accessible through Sister Linen. The door was always locked and she kept the key safely so that the flow of linen was regularly monitored and every item carefully checked. The linen was laid out alphabetically.

Sister Housekeeper was in charge of the domestic workers. She checked that these staff were on duty and dressed appropriately. The ward sister ensured that they conducted themselves properly and that the wards were clean. It was also the job of Sister Housekeeper to supervise the maids in the cleaning of the doctors' residence and the serving of their meals. It was Sister Housekeeper who would lead the long crocodile of girls in pink or green from the maids' home to the various hospital departments.

Sister Kitchen was responsible for all diets and for teaching trainee nurses general and invalid cooking as part of their training. She was also the dietitian. Here she managed the salt free, low calorie, diabetic and other special diets.

Without the administration sisters the system would have ground to a halt. These people ensured that the standards the matron wanted were rigorously adhered to. By the middle of the twentieth century administration sisters were responsible for all day-to-day running of the clinical areas. They would organize the holiday lists for the staff, and the allocation of nurses to wards, departments and educational activities. Every day there would be ward rounds, and these would be as thorough as matron's. Matron's rounds ended in the early 1970s, and when they did patients remarked how they missed the sense of security these visits to the ward had provided. The main purpose of the ward round was patient welfare and the monitoring of sound clinical practice, not only for the nurses but also for the medical staff. If there was any slackness in clinical procedures it would be picked up and dealt with immediately. These rounds could be intimidating for the staff, but were particularly noted for giving confidence to the patients. When a person in authority approached the patient or their relatives, they felt as if someone of importance was taking an interest in their well-being. It did not matter whether they thought it was the matron or not, it was authority.

There was a need for great flexibility among these sisters as they could expect to be asked to assist in any area when workloads required it. Working in the nurse administration office gave them a good insight into the general running of the hospital and a taste – or not – for further advancement. The most senior sisters would get a feel for the role of administration by being in charge of the whole hospital for an evening. Still running their own wards they had to go round the hospital resolving any problems. They could just as well be taking people to the mortuary as sorting out staffing issues. They did not get paid extra for this responsibility; they said that they were proud to do it.

Any problems in the wards, the maintenance department, the laundry, the kitchens and the chapel were reported directly to the matron's office. Even the mortuary was included to ensure that there was sufficient space for that day's bodies and that the flowers were always fresh. Where one ward was short an arrangement was made for another to help. Each evening there would be a matron's report to write on all new administration issues, new admissions and patients. This report was always given to the matron and shared with the night sister; hence the special knowledge of patients which always surprised nurses. As one matron said, 'I would even know if a patient had been admitted with a bad toe.'

Nurses well remember returning from sick leave and receiving a cool reception from the administration sister; nurses were not meant to be sick themselves. If they did not receive a lecture in the administration office they certainly got one when they arrived back on the ward. Many nurses would be told, 'You would not have been employed in my time. How do you think the patients can get well when the people who are supposed to look after them are going off sick themselves?' Invariably, the offending nurse would be sent to the sluice room for the rest of the day.

Margaret Webster suggested that the real dragons were probably found among the administration sisters, not the matrons. 'If we spoke to a medical student more than once we were sent to an annexe which was miles from our hospital in Sheffield. Here, there was only plastic surgery and neurology. You could spend nearly three years there, with no consideration for training needs.' With a rueful smile, she added, 'I know!' This annexe was a little isolated so the police often called. One night two policemen stayed a bit longer because the weather was so awful. During the night the roof started leaking and the following day it was discovered that the lead lining had been stolen during that night. As she said, 'We never did let on to the authorities about the policemen staying to escape the rain.'

Nurse administrators were undoubtedly worked hard, to the point where they could be too busy to take notice of their own health. An assistant matron of a north London hospital arrived home early one autumn morning in the early 1960s after suffering stomach discomfort in the night. She saw her teenage daughter off to school and should also have seen off her husband, a haematologist in charge of the hospital's blood bank, but she was feeling rather more tired than usual. She went upstairs to bed and asked her husband to bring her a cup of tea. On his way upstairs he heard her shout: 'Come quick, I think I'm about to have a baby!' Instructed by his wife he delivered a little boy and wrapped him in a towel. He then put the baby in the washing basket and rang their local doctor. He soon arrived, exploding with laughter. Neither she nor her husband had had any idea that this happy event was taking place. The new father then had to telephone the incredulous hospital to explain why the assistant matron would not be at work for the next few weeks and to ask whether he, too, could have a few days off to recover!

On promotion to an administrative post many sisters found they had lost something along the way. It was a sense of belonging and the ability to influence care directly. Ann Hirons, later the matron of Birmingham General Hospital, remembers:

> Moving from ward sister to the administration department I realized I had lost something that I had belonged to. It was not just the hands-on clinical work. As sisters, the responsibilities we had were enormous, and we had real influence, you could even knock the housemen into shape. For me ward sister was the most satisfying job in the hospital.

A major restructuring of nursing came in the early 1970s. Along with the post of Matron the role of the administration sister was no longer thought appropriate. Nurses were to be graded and the role of these sisters was taken over by nursing officers – a managerial role.

Some of the administration sisters were appointed and ward sisters promoted to these new posts, but many could not adapt to the changes and nursing lost many outstanding sisters.

6   Sister Tutors

I always believed that a tutor should spend time on the wards;
you could not sit in an office and hope to know what was
happening at ward level.

Margaret Watts, former sister tutor at
Farnborough Hospital, Kent

Before Florence Nightingale became involved with the training of
nurses, instruction was often insufficient to carry out the most basic
care practices. The nurses were poorly educated and the selection
processes almost non-existent. The Nightingale School at St
Thomas's Hospital, London, changed this situation and transformed
nursing.

Opened in 1860, the school was initially overseen by Mrs
Wardroper, the matron of St Thomas's Hospital, who was instrumental in introducing an improved quality of candidate for nurse
training. With the advent of Miss Crossland, a better-educated group
of nurses began working on the wards. Although primarily Home
Sister at St Thomas's Hospital, she also recognized the importance of
'taking classes', the forerunner of the role of Sister Tutor. In her
twenty-one years at St Thomas's Hospital, Miss Crossland played an
important role – it could be argued the major role – in advancing the
training provided to the probationers. She introduced a more organized system, with a consistent and complete schedule of training. In
her role as both home sister and teacher she was closely involved with
the development of both the nurse probationers and the special (lady)
probationers – the former had a more elementary instruction than the
latter. Both these groups needed direction, particularly with reading
lists. Initially a great deal of her time was spent supporting the poor

reading and writing abilities of nurse probationers. She would sit in at all lectures; she took comprehensive notes from the doctors and rewrote them with the probationers. She would diligently read the many notes they produced and correct any mistakes in content, grammar and spelling.

Most of the instruction had come from the medical staff but Miss Crossland increasingly took on the role of teaching them herself about a wide range of clinical matters, including the classification of medicines, their origin and their uses. There was also instruction in elementary anatomy and physiology, chemistry, poisons and their antidotes, weights and measures and reading prescriptions. The mornings were devoted to anatomy, physiology, hygiene, dietetics and invalid cooking. Writing to Miss Nightingale it 1876, she expressed her strong belief that 'Theory is very useful when carried out by practice', and that 'Theory without practice is ruinous to nursing'. So afternoons were devoted to more practical lessons: bandaging, bed-bathing and feeding helpless patients. Deeply religious, she was also enthusiastic about holding bible classes alongside her instruction. The nurses undertook a seven-week preliminary training, with a written examination at the end.

The standard training for nurses progressed rather more slowly than Florence Nightingale had envisaged, however. Apart from the Nightingale School there were very few hospitals offering training to new nurses either in London or the provinces. For many years following Nightingale's reforms, sisters and matrons at most hospitals were still essentially untrained and unable to give instruction in the most elementary tasks. There were very few nursing textbooks and the only available lectures were those from the medical staff – and these were few. New nurses were often expected to give enemas and dress wounds without any proper form of instruction.

This parlous and perilous situation provoked Rebecca Strong, Matron of the Royal Hospital, Glasgow, to complain in the *Nursing Record* in 1894 that there was no uniformity of education, general tests or examinations. In 1895 Isla Stewart, Matron of St Bartholomew's Hospital, wrote in a similar vein, pointing out the great variations in standards between different hospitals, some of which had preliminary training schools and others did not. Some of those that did used examinations, others did not. Some awarded certificates, others did not. Some offered a one-year, some a two-year, and some a three-year training course. But at the end, all could claim to be trained nurses.

These complaints are not surprising; teaching was not given high priority at many hospitals and infirmaries. In 1898, the guardians at the Fishpool Institution suggested an improvement in classes for the nurses. They were to be increased to once a fortnight from October to April inclusive. These classes were for the practice of bandaging and instruction in the principles of nursing, and to give instruction to the nurses and probationers in bedside nursing in different wards. The matron was to keep a record of all such instruction and the nurses' attendance. The report book of instruction was to be regularly checked by the medical superintendent.

One of the more successful preliminary training schools was at the London Hospital. It opened in 1895 and was named Tredegar House. Probationers from this school were known as the Tredegars. It usually took groups of thirty-two, with each of the new Tredegars being assigned a number. They were then known by these numbers throughout their initial training. At meal times they were marked in and had to sit according to their number at one of two long tables, with a sister presiding and saying grace. Breakfast was served at 7.00 every morning. This was followed by an hour's hectic cleaning in which the sister would literally stand over the probationers with a stopwatch while they carried out timed tasks such as bed-making, washing, sweeping and dusting before attending the training school. The subjects covered were elementary physiology, medical nursing, anatomy and surgical nursing. In 1901 a cookery kitchen for 'sick cookery' classes, where probationers spent some considerable tuition time, was added.

The beginning of the twentieth century saw a great advancement in the selection of nurses for training. The attributes of a nurse were by now quite exacting, as M.E. Fox explained in *How to Become a Nurse*.

Unselfishness, kindness, sympathy and patience, to be cheerful and pleasant in manner, for 'snappy' or sarcastic people, though they may become efficient, will not make lovable nurses. She must, above all things, be trustworthy – a real 'rock of defence' on whom her sick may lean in entire confidence – and she will also need plenty of 'grit' and perseverance to succeed in a very trying and difficult calling. If, in addition, a candidate is quick, quiet, self-controlled, cleanly and orderly in person and habits, adaptable and even-tempered, she is likely to make a very good nurse.

Before the First World War there was little change in the tuition of nurses; it still fell mainly to the home sister. It was 1914 before the first sister tutor or sister instructress, Miss Agnes Gullan, was appointed at the Nightingale School, St Thomas's Hospital. Outside London, one of the first sister tutors was Miss Durston, who was appointed to the Royal Hospital for Sick Children, Bristol, in 1922. Trained at the Middlesex Hospital she somehow managed to combine the role of Sister Tutor with that of Theatre Sister. For these burgeoning sister tutors a short course was introduced in 1927, but it was not until 1947 that the first examination for sister tutors was introduced following a one-year course; a two-year course started five years later.

Alice Ashworth, who trained at the Northern General Hospital in Sheffield in 1937, described the first time she saw the sister tutor.

There she stood, waiting for us at the top of the school steps arms folded; she was the sister tutor, and she did not look very agreeable. Short, thin, red-haired, and a little too stern for what we expected, but the more we got to know her, the more we found that she was ideally chosen for such a post. To be honest she seemed rather humourless for us young girls but we soon learned differently; and learn we did. She fed us knowledge like no one else; she also spent a lot of time talking about nursing life in her younger days, and our respect grew. The more she shared her own experiences, the more we wanted to nurse. This made it both interesting and fun. She did most of the teaching, with assistance from two junior sisters, but her classes were undoubtedly the most looked forward to.

In 1937 a block system of training was introduced at the University College Hospital, London, where Marjorie Houghton was the sister tutor. A nurse would have classes of theoretical instruction and then spend practical time on the ward. This new arrangement caused some exasperation among the ward sisters but was well received by the nurses; it was intended that the need to attend lectures after night duty or at other inconvenient times would end. Unfortunately the combined approach of theory followed by practice did not always go to plan; a nurse would often be rather haphazardly placed on a medical ward after learning the practice of surgical nursing or vice-versa. Pip Bradstock feels she has now seen student nurse training come full circle – 'not quite the earlier model but more in line with that than for the past many years'. Following the move to university education, with its high drop-out rate, there is now a move back almost to a block training system. Students are trained in groups with a tutor; they have a block of education then go to an area for practice, for example surgery, medicine or paediatrics. 'After all,' Pip said, 'nursing has always been and should be practice-based.' Prior to this change the sister tutor of the preliminary training school taught the nurses all the basics of nursing: how to make a bed, how to feed patients and how to bed-bath them. By the time the nurses went on to the wards they were fully prepared.

Jean Holland was very proud to have been taught by Sister Tutor Muriel Powell (later Dame Muriel Powell). A remarkable person, she was a perfectionist and a hard taskmaster, but it was thanks to this that Jean and her colleagues were happy to describe the training at Manchester Royal Infirmary as 'superb'. Her words rang in these nurses' ears throughout their careers. 'When I have done with you girls, you can work anywhere in the world and hold your heads up high because there will be no nurse better than you.' Jean emigrated to a successful career in America.

Muriel Powell's interest in nurse education continued throughout her extensive career. As Matron of St George's Hospital she made several changes in education at both hospital and national level, one of which was the forerunner of a graduate-level education for nurses through the introduction of a 'two plus one' course in 1966. This was a two-year theoretical course when the student would be supernumerary to the staffing complement, and one year in the clinical area to gain practical skills. A great innovator across education and clinical practice, she kept her feet firmly on the ground, and never lost her sense of fun and humour.

One of her duties as Sister Tutor at the Manchester Royal Infirmary was to teach medical students some basic nursing skills in just two lessons. The students tended to take these sessions very light-heartedly. Muriel was very attractive, which inevitably meant that at some point she was bundled into a bed as a practice patient. Nevertheless, the students had great respect for the nursing activities they were taught, including the intricacies of envelope corners for bed making.

Joan Jennings met Miss Powell much earlier in her career; both were in the same training set at St George's Hospital, London, and remained great personal friends until Dame Muriel's death on 8 December 1978. Joan remembers one of many incidents during their training.

One day in 1939 four of us held on to Muriel's legs when she was determined to lean out of a third-floor window to unfurl a banner. There was much laughter over this prank, with little thought to the dangers associated with hanging someone practically upside down. But that was typical of the determination she always showed.

Needless to say, each succeeding generation of student nurses played pranks with the equipment in the school. As a student nurse, Ann Hirons had great fun, both in the nurses' home and in the training school.

How Sister Tutor put up with us sometimes I do not know. So many times she would come into the class room and find 'Jimmy' the skeleton or the instruction model in all sorts of poses, even hanging out of the window, often with a cigarette dangling from its mouth.

Apart from 'Jimmy' the school would normally also have a bed with a life-size head and torso dummy, with a range of body parts. Since new nurses had no idea where these fitted, they would create great laughter among their colleagues by putting the wrong bit in the wrong place.

Joan Page, who retired as Matron of Kent and Sussex Hospital in 1970, was trained at Queen's Hospital for Children, Hackney Road, in 1942. 'There was no preliminary training school, or block system. Sister Tutor or the consultant physician who lived in the hospital during the war gave the lectures when they could. It was no problem to us, we just followed the excellent example of the ward sisters.' On the first day, the probationers attended in full uniform, with clean unrumpled aprons. The sister tutor's first words to them were, 'You must expect to be reprimanded while you are training, it is the way in which you will learn. The time to worry is when the sister does not tell you when you are not working well, because that will mean she does not expect you to improve.'

'I knew the truth of this when I became a sister,' said Joan. 'I had a student and completely gave up on her!'

Margaret Watts became interested in nurse education and training at the Miller General Hospital, Greenwich, believing that the fundamental purpose of nurse training was an investment of knowledge into the next generation so that nursing could develop. She was encouraged to go to Battersea College, London, to take a two-year diploma in nurse education. As a sister tutor she developed the greatest respect for the role of clinical teacher and the importance of the tutor's teaching at ward level. She felt that clinical teaching was of enormous benefit to the trainee nurse, and took a great deal of pressure off both the sister tutor and the ward sister, as both became more aware of the significance of each other's role. It also gave the education department an opportunity to see if any other teaching was taking place on the ward and provided a clear link between education and practice. Clinical teachers on wards would teach practical procedures linked to the teaching from the school. 'With this instruction of theory and practice taught in the school and the added confidence that this gives, they never lost the skill.'

When a nurse commenced training she was given a schedule of nursing procedures to be taught on her ward placement. The sister also had her own schedule of what she thought a nurse should have been taught by the time she left her ward. Here the trainee nurse learned what standards were. A sister would not mark a nurse competent in a procedure unless she showed that competence, and this was measured against the sister's own standards, which were far more demanding than the schedule.

When Joan Eddings was training at Westminster Hospital, she

found that hygiene was constantly referred to in the training school. 'It made a lot of sense,' Joan said. 'I felt that it prepared the nurses not only for the endless cleaning work on the wards, but for the importance attached to working with people who had wounds and were weakened through general ill health.' The nurses were taught the importance of hand-washing, food care, keeping a clean house and room, even cleaning drains. The message was the same: there were germs everywhere. 'We learned about micro-organisms on our skin, rats down drains, patients' locker surfaces covered with germs, instruments covered with bacteria, and that it was our fault if a patient got an infection while in our care; it meant that we had not taken sufficient care to clean and sterilize equipment properly.' The school was there to establish the basics of all the cleaning, wiping, polishing, disinfecting and sterilizing that was to dominate the nurses' lives on the wards. Cleanliness was inherent in nurse training, it was inherent in ward work; the whole ethic from Nightingale onwards was cleanliness. The instruction a nurse gained from the ward sister, sister tutor and matron was that cross-infection was a hazard to health and not to be tolerated.

Starting back at Queen Alexandra Hospital, Cosham, after a three-year break in America, Sylvia Kemp wanted to convert from state enrolled nurse (SEN) to state registered nurse (SRN). Matron De La Court was very proud of her SENs and was not too keen to lose them. Nevertheless Sylvia applied to take the entrance examination. Just scraping through, she then had to approach Matron De La Court. She was working with Sister Winters, who knew what Matron would say, and advised, 'Don't ask that old devil if you can do it, go and tell her you are going to do it!' Sylvia entered the office to be met by the matron leaning forward with her hands on her desk. 'Matron,' she said, 'I am going to do my state registration, I have passed the test.'

The response was: 'Yes I know, we must be scraping the barrel, you just got through.'

Nevertheless she was allowed to do her training.

Our clinical tutor was so pedantic about everything, especially grammar and spelling. It was almost as if the content did not matter as long as it was grammatically correct. We used to say, 'Have we got the answer right?' But it would come back, 'Don't tabulate nurse, never let me see you tabulate'.

Valerie Grey also found that her sister tutor was determined that the nurses would spell properly, 'She had no time for anyone who could not spell. It was more important than what the nurse had written.'

In 1950 Norma Clacey commenced a pre-nursing course. In the first year it was two-thirds education and one-third nursing; in the second year this was reversed.

We all failed because the school teacher did not appreciate the level of education required in a hospital; she was an ordinary teacher who taught biology; she did not have the background or knowledge to pass on to us as students. There was great anxiety as we were all hoping to go to the training school for our nurse training.

Matron De La Court nevertheless took them on and sent them to the school of nursing to learn how to pass the examination. She acquired an advance from their forthcoming wages to take it, and they all passed. As Norma said, 'I firmly believe it was the Sister Tutor's knowledge and training that brought us through. We learned to list facts rather than write compositions.' Later as a sister Norma taught practical skills on the ward.

I would have a student strapped up with a leg splint and then get the nurses to put them on the commode. Although it caused shrieks of laughter the nurses were more aware and more considerate of how patients felt. I had learned these practices from my sister tutor so it was common sense to pass them on in this way. I bet they would not do that to the modern student.

Wards were constantly monitored for their suitability for nurse training at specific intervals by a team from the General Nursing Council, later the English National Board, which then became the Nursing and Midwifery Council (NMC). Brenda Beech (née Crane) was a student on one such visit: 'As the inspectors moved from ward to ward so some of us were sent ahead of them to make it look as if there were more students on duty than there were. It must have quite baffled them at the large number of nurses who looked so alike.' The ward sister was pivotal to this learning process.

There were some die-hard attitudes from the past and some sisters found it hard to adapt. In these cases the weapon used to effect change was to threaten to take the ward out of training. Rightly or wrongly the sister could not do without student nurses – they were an integral part of her ward establishment. An area of concern was the allocation of student nurses to the wards. When training was ward based, ward allocation could often be carried out for the benefit of the system, not the learning needs of the students, so that allocation to learning areas could easily be manipulated, with trainee nurses being used to plug the gaps on wards.

There has always been an argument in nursing training over the balance between theory and practice. Was it weighted too heavily to one or the other? At ward level there was a similar issue over theoretical considerations and care practice. This was overcome for many years through the training of SENs. They had a two-year training and hospitals were more flexible with hours, which suited married women with family responsibilities. A good SEN would be highly prized. They were, however, taken advantage of and given more responsibility than they should have had. Many sisters rue the day when SEN training was abandoned. Here they had nurses who could take responsibility for the more practical aspects of care.

Pauline Ellison, who trained at St James Hospital, Portsmouth, had a view of traditional nurse education as that of an apprenticeship based on learning on the wards, backed up and supported by teaching input from the school of nursing. In this, the ward sister was always pivotal, in providing practical experience based on learned knowledge.

We probably were abused as students, but I did a hell of a lot of learning, from a combination of the sister tutor and ward sister. The theoretical approaches to practical aspects of our general training were good and obviously included subjects no longer taught. The sister tutor clearly related theory to practice, thinking things through, problem solving, and how treatment worked. Then we went to the ward and Sister took over.

The training of nurses has now undergone radical change from hospital-based to university-based. Many have expressed concern that the traditions of Nightingale have been lost. Said one sister, 'It is as if many of the basic values of our founder have been eroded. Do they teach these people about our traditional practices? The link seems to have been lost, along with the sister tutor and clinical tutor.' Another ward sister suggested that it should have been a refining process. 'Why am I still telling people to do simple things like mouth care, still having to remind them not to go off at meal times because there are people to be fed? These are such fundamental things, yet I am still having to remind new nurses to make the patient clean and comfortable.' Another complained, 'I have been around a long time battling on about mouth care. If teaching were the same surely we would not be chasing these basic care things would we? We were brought up when they were the day-to-day bread and butter of nursing.' Jacqueline Collett remarks:

> We used to take exams on how to bed-bath, how to feed someone, how to treat pressure sores, do they now? The whole emphasis was hands on, and the importance of caring and nurturing, these were important. But to be fair, they did not have the paperwork, the intravenous drugs, and the constant admissions; you could concentrate on that patient's care. It was routine, yes, but was it so wrong?

At the completion of training a nurse had gained theoretical and practical skills in the training school which they took with them for their ward experience; the art of nursing was learned on the wards from the ward team and the ward sister. On completion of this training at Westminster Hospital, Joan Eddings and her colleagues had already set their sights high. 'Now we had our certificates and hospital badge we thought we were ready to change nursing. What we all wanted was to get to the post of ward sister, because that was it, the person in that post could influence the care of the patients in any area of nursing.'

The world of education is changing fast. The Internet has meant that information is readily available to every nurse and rapid clinical changes mean that they must be continually prepared to update their knowledge. The qualification date was never an end to learning, and the best nurses were always those eager to enhance their expertise. Traditionally the sister tutor was the fount of all knowledge, but she has now been replaced by the university lecturer whose role is to develop skills of lifelong learning. 'The clock can never be turned back,' said one university lecturer, 'but there may be aspects of the old sister tutor and clinical teacher roles that we should have hung on to.'

7   Medical Ward Sisters

The very first requirement of a hospital is to do the sick no harm.
Florence Nightingale, *Notes on Hospitals*, 1863

Until Florence Nightingale's reforms hospitals were not healthy places to be nursed in. With virtually no understanding of infection control, lives were lost as infectious pathogens swept through the wards. Patients would die, not through their original illness but from fever that was endemic. Although there were fever hospitals, most medical wards accommodated an incompatible mixture of physically ill and fever patients, who would be nursed in the same open ward. The 1860s played host to smallpox, scarlet fever and typhus, which were rife in the community and consequently in hospitals. Doctors and nurses risked their lives daily, and many died. When Florence Nightingale returned from the Crimea she determined that these conditions would be tolerated no longer.

At first partitions were erected to separate the physically ill from the fever cases. Then fever patients were moved to upper floors before it was recognized that these people could not even be in the same hospitals as physically ill patients. It was the middle of the 1890s before most general hospitals were free of patients with contagious fevers. Even when Alice Ashworth began nursing at the Northern General Hospital, Sheffield, in the 1930s there were a lot of patients with pneumonia on the medical wards, as well as patients with typhoid fever.

We regularly nursed typhoid patients on the same ward as those with medical conditions and we were told that if we or the other patients contracted it, it would be our fault. We certainly learned what barrier nursing was. We nursed patients all the time, you never went past a patient without giving them a drink and cleaning their tongue. My goodness, sister would be on to you if you neglected anyone.

What was undoubtedly true, she pointed out, was that when pneumonia patients recovered they did so purely because of good nursing – there were no antibiotics.

At the end of the nineteenth century a probationer nurse was usually placed on a medical ward for her first experience in nursing. Under the watchful eye of the ward sister she learned the basics of care, basics that carried her through her nursing career. This training provided her with an introduction to the use of the clinical thermometer, giving an enema, making a bed, washing a patient, feeding and preventing bedsores. It also introduced her to cleanliness. One nineteenth-century sister thought the discipline of cleaning was a good one, and that it measured a nurse's suitability for her new role. She thought a nurse who found these tasks disagreeable would never make a good nurse.

It has always been recognized that some of a nurse's work is not exactly soul-stirring, and the sluice room dominated the junior nurse's life. This consisted of the instruments and bowl sterilizer, lavatories and the sluice itself. There were shelves for pot or glass bedpans and hooks with small towels for the bedpan covers. On the men's ward would be a row of pot or glass urinals. There would be large stone jars with a solution of carbolic made up by the nurses, holding large forceps. In the corner would be the soiled dressing bin. In the morning the routine for the medical ward sluice nurse was to collect all specimens of faeces, sputum and urine, then measure and label them and send them for investigation. She would drain, measure and clean Winchester bottles, clean sputum mugs, bedpans, and urine bottles and wash heavy rubber macintosh sheets and dry them on a special roller in the bathroom.

Every afternoon the sluice was cleaned thoroughly. The nurse would be provided with a rubber apron and if she was fortunate old surgical gloves. The instruments were washed and boiled in the sterilizer. Any soiled sheets had to be sorted and counted, checked by the sister, bundled up in a clean sheet and placed outside ready for collection. The most disagreeable jobs were the bedpan and sputum specimens, which were kept aside for inspection by the medical staff. When their contents were checked they had to be discarded, which could be a messy job. Then began the cleaning, disinfecting, and stacking on the racks. A routine day of cleaning was familiar to any nurse on a hospital ward until the 1970s. It was seen as the cornerstone of traditional ward work.

One morning a month would be locker morning. The lockers would be emptied, scrubbed and disinfected. The sister would check that the water was always hot and tell the nurse to go and change it if not. It might also be the patient's turn to gain the sister's disapproval if she spied something that should not be there, as Allen Gibbs nearly discovered when he was in hospital.

I was given a motoring magazine by one of the other patients to cheer me up. When I looked at it, it was just a cover for a rather naughty magazine hidden inside. Sister came out of her office so I quickly hid it in my locker. It happened to be the day sister chose to do her locker checking round. Fortunately she was not interested in cars!

Ward sisters managed their own ward maids and cleaners, and night sisters managed the 'scrubbers', who cleaned all the non-inpatient areas. They cleaned with little more than bare hands and a great deal of vigour; floors were scrubbed, sinks were scoured and brasses polished. Floor scrubbing was a speciality and an opportunity for the 'floor-scrubbers' to show off their skills, polishing, bumping and buffing until the floors shone.

Mary Verrier remembers that in the 1940s medical wards tended to be grim places with brown and green walls. Screens for privacy were constantly pushed up and down the wards, and few had wheels. After dinner the ward was effectively closed for an hour. Screens would be pulled across the door and peace would reign for the patients, but not for the nurses. The sister would instruct them to hand-make dressings and cotton wool swabs, then pack the drums for autoclaving and any other tasks she thought would fill a quiet hour.

Rubber gloves were repaired by pinching out a bit of rubber from an old pair and attaching it with a special glue. Bandages were also washed and ironed at this time. Mary added:

Baths for patients were at thermometer, not nurse's elbow, temperature. Mustard baths were one ounce of mustard for every gallon of water; we were good at guessing. For respiratory relief steam kettles (Allen) of hot water and friar's balsam or menthol crystals were used. The end of the bed had a wooden frame like a clotheshorse, draped with a sheet. It the patients became too moist and distressed you would transfer them to a warm, clean bed with clean, warm night garments.

Before the Second World War the sister's desk was normally in the centre of the ward, but it was later moved to the room at the end of the ward, when the sister no longer lived there. Here she would start her day. Following prayers she dealt with the paperwork and received the night nurse's report. At the table good deportment was essential: no shifting of feet when a nurse was tired, no part of the uniform untidy, no slovenliness. The sister had command of the whole ward and woe betide a junior doctor if he was caught writing notes there. From there she would also do her very detailed round of the patients. At each bed she would note the information on the charts, the condition of the patient, and any changes that had not been noted. She would also hand out the post. Through this routine she was in constant contact with the patients, fulfilling Florence Nightingale's belief that frequent contact between sisters and the patients was highly desirable. Following this the kitchen, the bathroom and the sluice room would be inspected.

Each day the sister or the senior nurse would allocate jobs to the nurses. The most junior would be responsible for giving out bedpans, helping patients on and off the commode or walking them to the lavatory, and doing the basic cleaning of tables, lockers and the sluice room. She soon learned to stow away equipment in an orderly fashion, and not leave the linen room untidy. The third-year trainee nurse usually did the daily urine testing, some of which required additives or the boiling of a small amount of urine in a test tube. The more experienced nurse would check and record the pulse, temperature and respiration of every patient. A qualified nurse would be responsible for any dressings, treatments and the medicine round.

Sisters were rightly fastidious about their record books, which continued in use on many wards until recent years. The information in them centralized the knowledge of the patients' conditions. In the bowel book would be recorded the daily habits or problems of the patients, so that their needs were unlikely to be overlooked at busy times. Also in the bowel book would be the daily allocation of enemas. Peter Bartlett was a patient in Victoria Ward, Royal Hants County Hospital, Winchester, in 1957 when he was involved in the classic retort to Sister Mumford's question: 'Good morning patients, have you all had your bowels open?' This was met by a chorus of 'Yes sister, have you?'

Integral to the focus on bowels was the bedpan round. Opening bowels and using bottles to order was no mean feat, but the patients were often expected to perform this task with the nurse hurrying to get the offending material out of the way before the consultant's round. Any patient who requested a bedpan during the round would not be regarded in a very good light. A nurse who carried only one or two bedpans at a time would not be too popular either. The expectation was that an experienced junior nurse should manage three or four at a time, and carry them the length of the ward. In the days when they were made of porcelain they would break when dropped and the later metal bedpans would make an infernal noise.

Alongside the bowel book would be the bath book and depending on the routine of a particular ward or hospital, patients would have a daily or weekly bath. The bath book recorded not only the frequency of baths but also the patients' skin condition. Where patients were incapable of having a bath, a bed-bath would be given. Bed-bathing was always done in a certain way: face, arms, legs, trunk and back. With young men the nurses were taught how to use the sheets so the patient was not unnecessarily exposed; the ones who were usually embarrassed were the young ones. Where possible the patients would be given a cloth to do the more intimate bits themselves. All pressure areas were treated thoroughly twice a day, and in the case of prolonged bed care at least four-hourly. For backs talc and surgical spirit were used liberally. The base of the spine, elbows, heels and hips were massaged by the palm of the hand, first with soap and water, then with surgical spirit and finally dusted with talcum powder. Nurses felt this was one of the fundamentals of care and a good opportunity to interact with the patients. Many nurses had questions about bedsores in their hospital examination but complained that they had never seen one.

The diet book would be updated daily in consultation with the medical staff. Diets were an integral part of the sister's role before the advent of the dietitian. On the medical wards there would be patients with diabetes and with stomach, liver and cardiac problems. Before the advent of kitchen supervisors the kitchen or administration sister would be responsible for the preparation of any diets requested by the ward sister; on the wards where this service was not provided, the nurses would prepare diabetic, low-calorie, fat-free and other diets.

Breakfast and dinner times were always important events, in many respects sister's speciality. She would preside over these occasions like a hawk; woe betide the nurse who gave out the wrong diet. The sister was in charge of the meal trolley and ensured that her patients had the food that was due to them. She directed the proceedings, and for many years the serving of meals carried great status. In this way she got to know who was and was not eating and who could eat a large meal. It someone required something more delicate, she would provide an alternative. She could also direct nurses to assist patients who were not eating. However, serving meals brought out the eccentricities of one sister where Marion Dyson trained.

When we were very busy, the sister used to completely forget what she had taught us. She would hand us a plate of food and say, 'Take that to the leg (thrombosis)', or 'Take that to the appendix.' If we had said that she would have gone mad; I am sure she did not know she was doing this. But through her I learned the importance of sister being there when meals were served. She would say, 'Nurse, it is common sense that an ill patient will push a meal away, it is also common sense to find out why.' Cups of tea were given out after the meal was over. 'You would not give someone a cup of tea until they have finished their meal, would you?' she insisted.

Bed-making was quite a skill, and there would be annual competitions between wards and hospitals at fund-raising fêtes. Dave Hurst's first experience of bed-making in a general hospital made him realize what an accomplished art it was. 'I thought it was a bit like my hobby, motor racing. An art of speed, dexterity and precision cornering.' Counterpanes had to show off any hospital motto in the centre of the bed, the open end of the pillow-case had to face away from the ward entrance, sheets were turned down to a regulation length, usually elbow to wrist, and wheels were turned in. Nothing in the school of nursing could prepare a new nurse for this. With experience a thirty-bed ward would take two skilled nurses less than an hour to complete. The patients would be aware of the work involved and would remain as stiff as ramrods in their beds lest they disturb the pattern of counterpane and sheet angle until the matron did her round. Dave Hurst's busiest day was when he accompanied the sister bed-making on an admission day. 'She included a teaching session would you believe it? I found it an exhausting experience, but Sister was just as fresh as when we started.'

Beryl Varilone remembered that in the middle of the ward at Devizes District Hospital was a large rectangular piece of furniture with drawers and cupboards on all four sides, called the stack. It was used to store drugs, instruments, spare linen, flower vases, and many more items. It was also the dining table for patients who were able to sit out. When patients were admitted they were seated on a chair beside the stack, newspapers were placed under the chair and a towel wrapped round the patients' shoulders. In full view of everyone their hair was combed with the nit comb to check for lice. If there was a problem they would then have their hair shampooed with Durback soap and some other foul-smelling substance such as sassafras oil. There they would sit with their heads wrapped in towels for some considerable time. During the Second World War in London nurses would regularly comb each other's hair at night as lice were so common from people having to sleep in the Underground during the bombing raids. The London hospitals were also overrun with cockroaches, mice and rats as a result of the bombing.

Visitors would often leave flowers, which were thought to eat up 'nocturnal' oxygen in the wards at night. This was deemed to be detrimental to the patients' health, so all flowers were removed before the night staff took over and taken out to the sluice room. It was the sister's job to return them to the ward in the morning. In this process she always did an initial round of the patients. Many sisters were so keen on their flower arrangements that no one was allowed to touch them. For one patient this caused a slight problem. The sister carefully prepared her jug of water and placed it on a table near the flowers, ready to top them up. She saw a nurse doing something wrong, which distracted her. On returning she found there was no water in the jug, 'Where has my water gone?' she demanded. A rather sheepish male patient replied, 'Sorry, Sister, I drank it.'

Daphne Fallows (née Bunney) explained how her liking for medical nursing developed at St Thomas's Hospital. For her this was more interesting as the focus of care was on the physiological rather than the anatomical; as she said, 'I never was very good with the skeletal system.' She thought medical wards were where real nursing was carried out and in this speciality the nurse got to know the patient better. In other areas of nursing she felt there was such a fast turnover on the wards that a nurse hardly had time to get to know the patient before they were gone. A great influence on her was the first occasion she worked with the sister on a bed-bath, 'a terrifying experience'. But the more the sister showed her, the more her respect grew. 'The patient was critically ill.' Daphne said. 'By the time we had finished half an hour later this same patient was smiling and talking.' Somewhat inexperienced, it was difficult for her to work out what the sister had done, but she had spent equal amounts of time on the bed-bath and on talking to the patient. 'I said to sister that it was a miracle that I had just seen. She replied, "No it was not, it was experience, but it takes many years to work in that way, and never forget it in your career."' She never did. That sister became her role model and medical nursing her main interest.

Coming directly from her psychiatric training, Pauline Ellison's first week in St Thomas's Hospital was the first time she had any real contact with a sister in a general hospital, and she was a sister with a formidable reputation. It was also the first time she saw a cardiac arrest. Fortunately there was a senior nurse and she and the sister went to deal with the situation until the support staff arrived. The sister dialled the emergency number and another nurse smashed the covering of a small box to remove a key to release the emergency trolley. The staff nurse went scurrying to get the box with the emergency medical equipment and the Ambu respirator. The patient's airway was checked and then the mask was placed over his mouth. By now the anaesthetist had arrived. In the drama that was unfolding Pauline did not know what to do.

So I thought, I know, I'll make a cup of tea for the other patients. When it came to pouring the tea out I was so high on adrenalin that the cups rattled as I gave them to the patients. When it was all over I was still in a state of shock and emotion, but Sister said, 'Very well done, nurse, the tea was very thoughtful of you, the patients appreciated it.'

From that moment she grew to respect the sister and with this her fearsome reputation faded.

When she was a student nurse on a medical ward Wendy Carson found the sister somewhat strict – so much so that even the male patients were wary of her. She still had inflexible rules for the ward, even when she was off duty. These included the fact that the main ward lights had to be turned off at 8.00 p.m. and the over-bed lights by 10.00. The sister would leave the ward at 8.00 after she had checked that the nurses had turned off the main ward lights but would sometimes come back during the evening. The men liked a game of cards, but when the sister was on duty she would not allow card playing. So as soon as she left the ward, the lights would go on again and out would come the cards. This was not as brave as it seems; they always posted someone near the main ward door just in case.

For her first ward allocation at the Royal Free Hospital, London, in 1965, Wendy Wild felt she was lucky to be placed on a medical ward. Many of the patients were old hands and had been admitted before, especially in the winter when their bronchitis was bad and their homes were cold and damp, so they knew the ropes and were a great help to an inexperienced student. It was on this ward that Wendy met her first death. Sister asked her if she wanted to help with the last duty a nurse had to patients, 'laying them out'.

This was quite different then. We nurses washed the whole body and packed the orifices. The patient was then dressed in a nightgown her relatives had requested. This was all done with

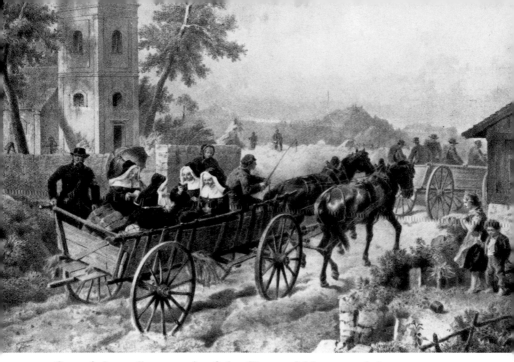

One of the earliest records of the Sisters of Mercy on their way to a battlefield to tend the wounded. This shows them during the Austro-Prussian War of 1866

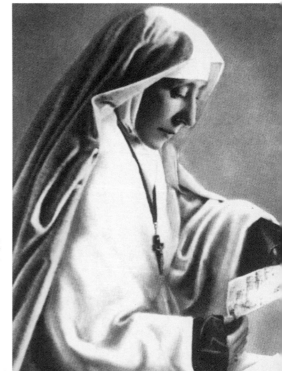

The Venerable Mary Potter, founder of the Little Company of Mary Sisters, 2 July 1877

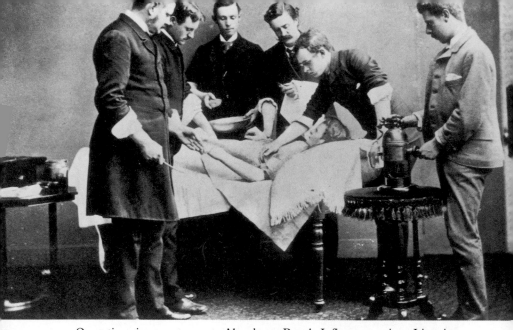

Operation in progress at Aberdeen Royal Infirmary using Listerian antiseptic methods, 1869. There were no masks, gloves, gowns or theatre sister

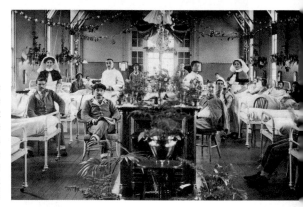

QAIMNC and male orderlies with the Blue Boys during the First World War. The service patients were always known by this name because of the issue of the blue uniform while in hospital

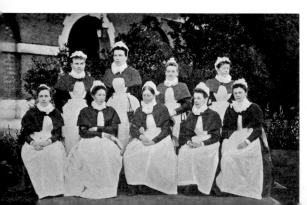

Head Sister Louisa Hogg and the small group of nursing sisters at Haslar Hospital, 1897

Sister Matron Eve Opie, of King's College Hospital c. 1952, was the last to be known by this title

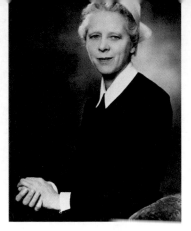

Staff and patients during the Christmas season on A1 ward at Milton (St Mary's) Hospital, Portsmouth, December 1912

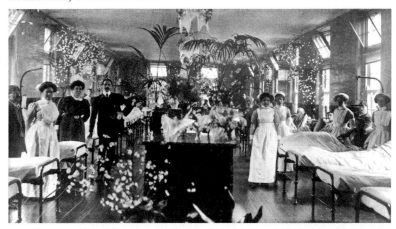

Matron A.B. Baillie and ward sisters at Bristol Royal Infirmary, 1906

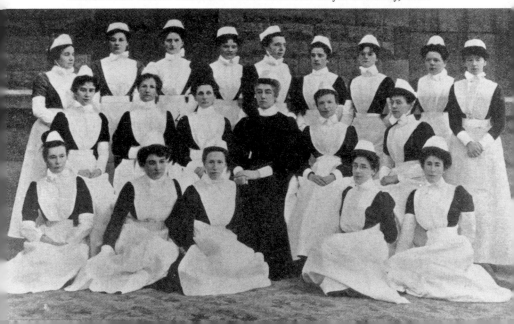

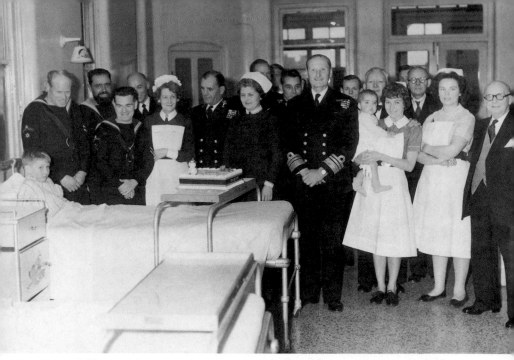

Officers and men of the Royal Yacht on their annual Christmas visits to the children's wards with one of the Christmas cakes baked while they were at sea, *c.* 1960

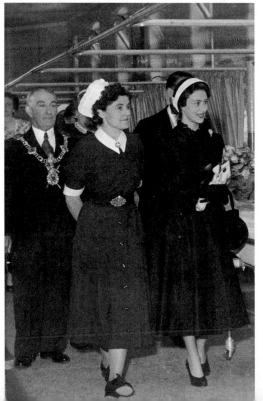

Royal visits were always popular with both staff and patients. HRH Princess Margaret on one of her regular visits to the Royal Hospitals, Portsmouth, escorted by Sister Millie Eldridge, 1952

Lucy Simon (later Baird) setting off on one her daily visits when district nurse at Euxton, Chorley, 1941

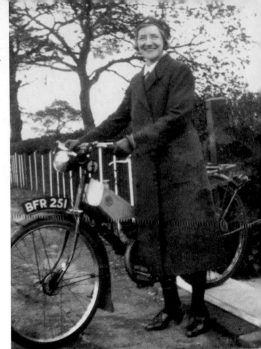

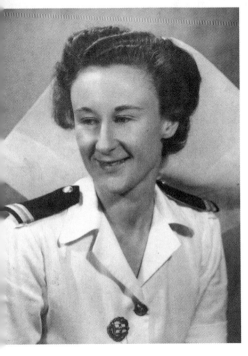

Billie Bisland (later Cullen) in the nursing sister uniform of the Orient Line travelling between the UK and Australia, *c.* 1950

Bella Keech (later Blandford) and Muriel Watkins (later Bright) in the midwives' outdoor uniform during their training at St George's Hospital, London, 1950

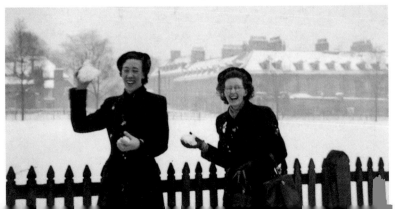

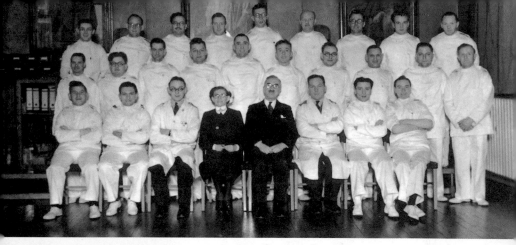

Reg Commander (*front row, second right*) and Don Bentley (*front row, second from left*) with Matron Gray, and Mr Cockburn, the house governor, Wolverhampton Royal Hospital, 1947

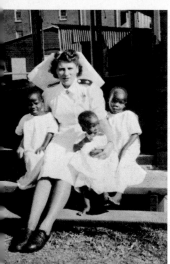

Margaret Watts with three child patients at King Edward VIII Hospital, Congella, Durban, *c.* 1950

John Greene (*second row, third from left*), one of a group of psychiatric nurses recruited for duty in naval hospitals and hospital ships, July, 1940

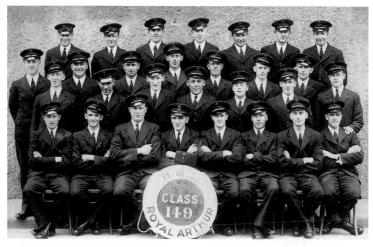

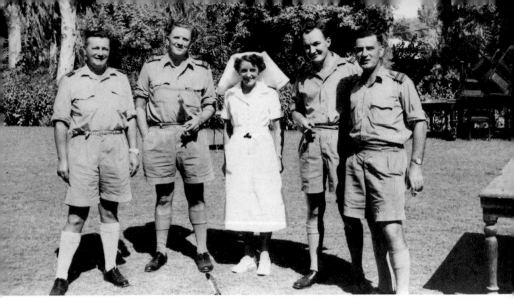

Flight Officer Mary Ellis (later Wrangham) *centre*, with (*left to right*)
Wing Commander Beer, Norman Hudson (dental), Tom Forrest
(anaesthetics), Paddy Ryan (stores), Baghdad, 1956

Matron De La Court (*centre*) and Sister Tutor Miss Bevan (*third from
left*) both Guy's Hospital trained, uphold the Guy's tradition of wearing
ties on prizegiving day at Royal Hospital, Portsmouth *c.* 1950

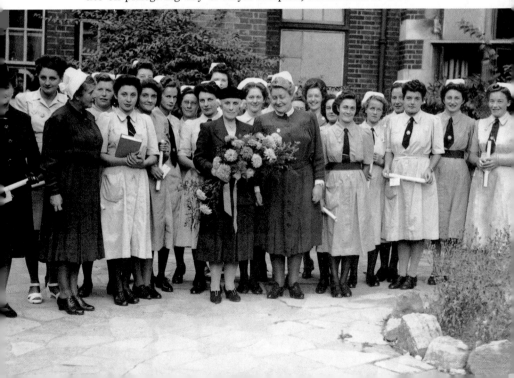

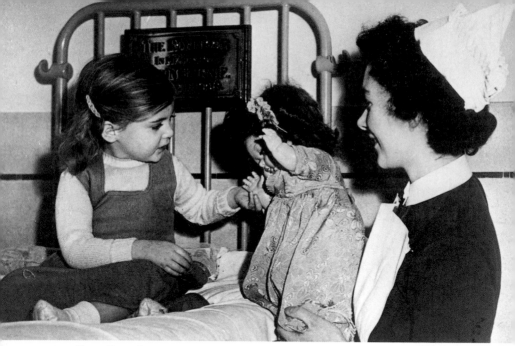

Sister Joan Page handing a Christmas present to a patient at the Royal
Free Hospital, *c.* 1956

Margaret Morris and fellow sisters energetically perform the can-can at
the Christmas show, Rush Green, 1958

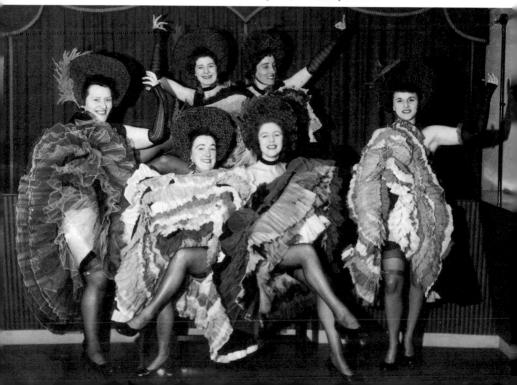

the greatest respect. Sister was very gentle both with the patient and with me, sending me for various articles when she thought I might be feeling upset. Although extremely busy, Sister was clearly aware that this was still her patient until removed to the mortuary.

These same principles applied to another patient on the ward. She was a girl of twenty-eight who had five children and was dying of heart disease. One afternoon shortly before she died, she was breathless, hot and uncomfortable. The sister arranged for the nurses to wheel her out into the sunshine with everything that she needed. The bed was taken out – oxygen cylinders, drips, everything. It took a number of nurses to get her on to the balcony. 'But it was worth it to see the patient so happy, it was part of the human face of nursing. She influenced me more than anybody; it was she who made me want to stay in nursing. Her whole life was to make the patients comfortable.'

'Medical wards were hard work,' remembers Tom Noakes, who trained at the Royal Hospital, Wolverhampton.

You never stopped, there were forty patients on a ward and you did everything. Insulins, fractional test meals [designed to eliminate gastric juice activity] treatments, back rounds, everything. They were the good old days of nursing, but not for patients; they died of illnesses that would be treatable now. I had a patient with progressive arteriole occlusion; this meant that little arteries would block, the tissue in the area would then rot causing those parts of the body extremities to die, requiring amputation of the limb. We just had to watch while his legs and his arms, one after the other were removed. It all went on for many months; there was nothing that could be done.

Barbara Hare, who trained at Bolingbroke Hospital, Clapham Junction, in 1954, also looks back with great sadness at the lack of treatment. Nephritis, a curable disease of the kidney today, killed. She remembers a young boy in end-stage renal failure. 'The only thing we had to help him were magnesium-sulphate enemas. That was all there was, there was no other treatment in those days, so all we could do was nurse him while he was dying. We just had to watch him die.'

Cardiac patients were treated with the only drug available, Coramin, and a patient would spend weeks of complete bed rest being moved only for their toilet needs, without any exertion on their part but a great deal for the nurses.

Pneumonia, stomach and duodenal ulcers, along with heart disease and kidney disease were the more common illnesses on medical wards of the 1960s. For a patient with congestive cardiac failure medical treatment consisted mainly of Digoxin, diuretics and antibiotics. Nursing care was aimed at giving the patient complete physiological rest, absolute stress-free rest with no unaided movement. The patient would be washed and fed. Oxygen was administered, the bowels kept open, a salt-free and low-protein diet given and pressure points dealt with half-hourly. As Joan Eddings pointed out, 'These patients responded to the basics of good nursing care; the traditionally trained nursing staff were geared to this.'

One of the major diseases throughout this period was tuberculosis (TB). Audrey Jones was trained in the care of TB patients at Elswick Hospital, near Preston. As she said, 'The patients were there for fresh air, and fresh air was what they got.' TB was prevalent in bad housing and overcrowded areas, so the aim was to give the patient clean air and space, and the only place for this was out of doors. The worst job she found was dealing with the sputum.

But we did do some very interesting work. We were taught how to stain the bacillus and observe it under the microscope once a week. From that we could see if the bacillus was still active. We had patients in the 1940s who had been prisoners in Germany, Japan and in the concentration camps, where conditions were ideal for TB. Unfortunately by the time they came to us it was too late and most patients died. I remember one whole family dying because the father, a major in the army, had been a prisoner of war and had passed on the bacillus to his wife and then to the daughter before it was diagnosed.

These TB patients had little in the way of medication, so when they did start to recover it was a slow process, one stage at a time. They would spend one hour in a chair by their beds, which was increased until eventually they had sat out for a full eight hours. Then they were allowed to walk about the sanatorium. Not being allowed to drink, they used to get 'unofficial' bottles of beer from the NAAFI, as well as other goods, but the medical superintendent could withhold this privilege if there were any infringements. Audrey explained:

One day the farmer of the field attached to the sanatorium complained that he could not work his field because of all the beer bottles. Sister went to deal with the complaint. When she got back she announced that there were hundreds of empty bottles in the field. It seemed the men drank their beer and when they finished they threw their empty bottles from their windows. They were detailed to go out and collect them; nearly 800 bottles were recovered. They were deprived of their beer 'rations' for a week.

Joan Jenkins worked in a sanatorium near Sheffield, where the patients slept on a cold balcony all night and the night nurses had to refill their stone hot water bottles every two hours in the winter. At 4.00 a.m. the beds were pulled back into the covered area, and at 5.00 a.m. the nurses started to wash the patients. After the patients had had their breakfasts they would immediately be pushed outside again. Some could even make fun of this. Tommy Cather was a patient who had been called up for the duration of the war. He was captured in Germany and sent to a concentration camp. There he contracted advanced bilateral TB. On the ward he would be seen every day with a crochet hook and different coloured balls of wool. Audrey said:

We would ask him what he was doing but he would not tell us. He would smile the unique smile of someone with an emaciated face and very large eyes. One day he would be using blue wool, another day yellow, so it went on. On Christmas Day we went to give the patients their breakfast, and they all had different coloured nosebags tied to their faces.

Margaret Morris was a sister at a respiratory unit at Romford Hospital in the 1950s at the height of the polio epidemic. There was a 26-year-old patient called Heather, who was paralysed from the

99

neck down, one of a few who did not have a tracheotomy. She was one of the first patients to be offered treatment in the tank respirator (the iron lung), which was first invented in America by Phillip Drinker in 1926. After being taught 'frag breathing', a special way of swallowing air, this machine gave her some independence. One day she announced that she would like to visit St Paul's Cathedral. She and a third-year nurse set off from Romford by train using parcel lifts instead of stairs to Liverpool Street station. At the bottom of the steps to the cathedral two men volunteered to carry the wheelchair, and the patient up the steps. After a delightful circuit of the cathedral they were again assisted down the steps. Problem number three came when hunger took over. Heather could not eat sitting up and 'frag breathing'. Once again someone came to their rescue, helping to get her out of the chair. On their return to the hospital it was agreed that it had been a wonderful time.

Heather was not finished, however. She decided that she wanted to visit her father in Belgium. He was a colonel in the army based in Antwerp. Although Margaret Morris offered to train two private nurses to escort Heather, she would not hear of it. She wanted Margaret and another sister to accompany her. Between them they organized two weeks' leave, and with her father's co-operation they took her to Antwerp. They travelled by freight air from Southend Airport with thirteen pieces of luggage. An ambulance, two orderlies and a doctor met them. It proved to be a very successful family visit. Heather had proved how determined she was and this determination was part of her life; she became a well-known foot and mouth artist and died in 1995 at the Lane Fox Respiratory Unit, St Thomas's Hospital, London.

The polio epidemic meant many fever wards had to be reopened. At Bromwich Fever Hospital, Birmingham, Tom and Alice Carr remember wards full of patients in iron lungs, mostly women and children, as polio was then known as the killer of young men. A man would go to a football match one week, mixing in the crowds, and be dead the next. There was no treatment. As a student nurse, Aileen Gardner was working on the medical ward when the first iron lung was introduced to St Mary's Hospital in Portsmouth in 1956. Sadly the very first patient who needed it was her own aunt, Jean Taylor.

In the early 1960s attention focused on the care of cancer patients and the care of the dying. Dr Cicely Saunders prepared the ground not only for the opening of St Christopher's Hospice in London, but also for the start of the hospice movement throughout the country. However she was not the first to open a hospice. In Ireland Mary Aikenhead of the Sisters of Charity (see chapter 1) founded Our Lady's Hospice for the care of the dying in Dublin, and in London the St Joseph Hospice was opened in the East End at the turn of the twentieth century. There were many other institutions and homes for the care of the dying, run mainly by religious orders, the exception being the Marie Curie Memorial Foundation. In 1980 there were over sixty hospices in Britain, and now these hospices had captured the interest of nurses and the support of the public. At one time, however, cancer care and the care of the dying were not very popular areas of work for nurses. They were usually seen as low-skill areas with little possibility of advancement. It is to Cicely Saunders's eternal credit that she changed the whole focus of cancer care. Where patients more often entered a hospice in a terminal condition, now they would more likely attend as an out-patient for pain relief and support long before terminal care. As a consequence, in recent years it has become a popular though still exacting speciality.

Another service that struggled for popularity was care of the elderly. For many years they were nursed in the old workhouse infirmaries. They were large institutions, and the care was mainly custodial. The patients handed over their belongings when they entered and would not see them until they were discharged (an unlikely event), so they were rarely dressed in their own clothes. As one nurse said, 'I worked in a geriatric ward for eight years and never saw patients dressed in their own clothes.' Cot sides on the beds were the norm and those few who were allowed up were often in restraint seats or tied with sheets in the chairs. One sister on a geriatric ward was full of good intentions, and was concerned about relatives drawing and misspending her patients' pensions. So every Wednesday she would organize a coach and 'her men' would be taken out. The nurses described it as a nightmare. She would go to the coach and cover the seats with incontinence pads. The nurses would be loaded up with urine bottles and vomit bowls, and the patients would be humped and bumped out of the ward and up into the bus. Most of them immediately fell asleep with their knitted blankets wrapped round them. Sister would not expect them back until 5 p.m. They would be taken somewhere local, hustled off the bus, bought a cake and a cup of tea, and put back on the bus. By the time the nurses got them back in the ward they were exhausted. Sister would cheerily say, 'Now you did enjoy that boys didn't you?' She never expected a reply, so she was not disappointed when there was none.

The 1970s saw a more selective approach to the individual needs of patients and nurses devoted to this type of care, but there was still a problem with age prejudice and lack of resources. However, along with new consultant geriatricians and psychogeriatricians the care of the elderly has undergone major changes with the introduction of a person-centred philosophy, specialist nurses and community care.

Jacqueline Collett continues to believe that for a medical ward there was a lot of sense to the Nightingale system.

The acute patients were nursed nearest the office, the less ill in the middle of the ward and those waiting to go home at the end. I know there was a cost to privacy but nurses could observe the acutely ill patients properly, and the nursing staff immediately knew who needed the most attention. The ones now who are potentially occupying beds are the desperately ill who need loads of help and cannot be discharged because there is nowhere to discharge them to. So you get a large majority who are desperately ill and need good, old-fashioned care.

8 Surgical Ward Sisters

To be Sister of a ward, where the hearts of her patients do safely trust her, and where she feels herself the trusted colleague of her Surgeon or Physician – that is happiness indeed.

> Isla Stewart, 'Practical View of Nursing',
> *Murray's Magazine*, 1890

The first of a long line of sisters on surgery wards were appointed in the late 1880s. It was a time when post-surgical care was becoming a specialist engagement for nurses. Prior to this there had been no recognition that surgical cases required anything but bed rest to recover. Those patients who did survive the shock of major surgery without an anaesthetic would have months of agonizing recovery. To add to the patient's discomfort would have been the changing of wound dressings. Until the advent of the Nightingale nurses, doctors and medical students always undertook this task; in this they were known as 'the dressers'. Unusually, in 1820 the Royal Devon and Exeter Hospital allowed its nurses to be involved with dressings, but only in fetching tins of warm water with which the doctor cleansed the wounds. They were allowed to apply either a bread or a linseed poultice, but as soon as other dressings were ordered, the medical pupil would take charge. If the patient's physical state was such that someone had to sit with them at night it was again the medical pupil who did this, not the nurse. It was also the doctor who took patients' temperatures; woe betide a nurse who was caught doing it, even under instruction from the doctor. Indeed, the secretary of St Mary's Hospital, London, would not permit the sisters or nurses to take temperatures, pulse beats or respiration rates at all.

Until the middle of the nineteenth century infection was thought to be part of the normal process in the mechanism of wound repair following an operation, so patients could be kept in bed for two or three months until healing occurred. Because of the lack of understanding of sterilization methods, many wounds did not heal adequately and the patient would be left crippled. The development of Lister's aseptic principles in 1865 changed the whole technique of surgical intervention. With the widespread use of carbolic spray in the operating room and the application of carbolic-soaked dressings to the wound, and aseptic techniques to prevent further introduction of bacteria, the first battle for 'clean' surgery and wound care commenced. At this time, however, Lister himself did not understand that prolonged scrubbing of hands was essential, not just washing them in carbolic then rinsing them in water.

In 1881 Doctor Willett, the surgeon at St Thomas's Hospital, lecturing to nurses on wound care informed them: 'There are three modes of healing: the first, most to be desired, but never seen, by first intention; the second, by granulation; the third, always seen and least desired, by suppuration [the discharge of pus from a wound].' Post-surgery patients were also prone to erysipelas, an acute streptococcal infectious disease of the skin characterized by fever, headache, vomiting and purplish raised lesions, particularly on the face. With the constant itching associated with the lesions it was not surprisingly also known as St Anthony's Fire. Wounds would have been treated with kaolin, mustard, laudanum, tincture of opium or poppy heads (which contained opium). The sister would prepare this poultice by using three or four poppy heads to one pint of water. Breaking them up she would discard the seeds and boil the rest in water for twenty minutes, strain and make a linseed-based poultice. Another popular poultice of the time was charcoal, because of its neutralizing effect on the objectionable smell from wounds where gangrene was present.

In contrast to the modern throughput of surgical patients, even the simplest operations required a lengthy recovery time. Patients were either laid flat or propped up in their beds with a firm 'donkey' pillow under their knees for days or weeks on end. Operations considered straightforward today were certainly not before the 1970s. For example, hernia repair required a prolonged recovery with possible complications. The patient would be starved the night before the operation then given an enema. In the morning he would be prepared for theatre by being washed from the waist down and shaved by the hospital barber, then clothed in a gown and bed-socks. During the operation the bed would have been prepared with a large cradle, often fitted with high-powered bulbs to keep the bed warm, in order to counteract shock. On return from theatre, noted Kay Riley, 'there was no post-operative recovery area; the surgical sister received the unconscious patients back from theatre and looked after them on the ward with all the other patients. Hence the benefit of the Nightingale ward with its easy observation.' The patient would face a one- to three-week period of lying completely flat and would only be considered fit to go home after another two weeks. Even then a period of convalescence followed.

A patient suffering from a peptic ulcer would now receive medication from a general practitioner and there would be a very good chance that no surgical intervention would be required. In the 1950s the most common treatment was a gastrectomy (the excision of part or the whole stomach). Pre-operatively it would normally involve passing a Ryle's tube (a thin weighted rubber or plastic tube) into the stomach. Post-operatively it would require a very lengthy stay in bed. It was at this point that the principles of basic nursing care came into play. The pulse would be taken every fifteen minutes and the blood pressure every half-hour. With pressure points being so vulnerable particular attention would be given to them. When consciousness returned the patient would then require the slow introduction of fluids via the tube and later by mouth.

As a trainee nurse, Ruth Sanders developed an enormous respect for a surgical ward sister at St Thomas's Hospital, who required that every job was to be carried out without shortcuts. Clearly the patients came first and every task was carried out with meticulous care.

After abdominal operations the patients would be on restricted hourly fluids. This was little more than sips of water. They were measured out exactly and kept in the fridge. When needed they would be taken from the fridge, put on a saucer, then on a tray and then taken to the patient. At the time I thought it was a little daft, but it was all the water they could have and Sister was

105

determined that it would still be something special for that patient. This was just one example where she saw to it that her patients had the best of care.

Joan Jenkins, who trained at St George's Hospital, also remembered a sister on the surgery ward. 'She ensured that every day each patient was bed-bathed. No patient could get up for at least ten days after an operation, but Sister ensured that everyone looked forward to the pleasure of those moments of individual attention.'

This sister also showed her the value of using common sense in an otherwise potentially difficult situation. One of the nurses had eaten some ice cream meant for the patients. Eating on the ward was strictly forbidden, and a dismissal offence. The sister came in one day and said, 'We are missing a number of ice creams, would anyone know about this?' One of the student nurses said, 'It must be the mice sister.' Sister replied, 'They must be big mice, and I suppose they will stop raiding the patients' food now, won't they?' She knew it would stop, and did not have to say anything more.

It was an unwritten rule for many years that under no circumstances was a nurse ever to give patients their Christian names. This rule was often flouted, and one day, on the way to the operating theatre the patient asked a nurse her name and she told him. Of course, surgical ward patients returned from theatre having had an anaesthetic. When he came round, the patient immediately asked for the nurse by name – in the presence of the ward sister. The nurse was greatly shocked when she was called to the sister's office and given a severe dressing down.

Marion Dyson (née Upson) was in her fourth year as a student nurse at Huddersfield Royal Infirmary when she was on night duty on a surgery ward. It was also her duty to scrub up as theatre nurse and assist the consultant. One night she had to prepare the theatre for two emergencies, including a ruptured spleen. When they were over she only had the assistance of one porter to clean up the theatre. As she was the senior student on the surgical ward it was also her responsibility to write the report for the day sister. Since she had been in theatre, she did not know anything about any of the patients on the ward that night, so she asked one of the nurses who had spent all night on the ward to write the report. The sister was very unhappy and pointed out to Marion that it was not a sufficient excuse to say that she had been busy in theatre.

Kay Riley recognized as a student nurse that she was more interested in the anatomical rather than the physiological workings of the body, and this she feels led her into the surgical branch of nursing. She also found it satisfying that surgery patients were discharged earlier, and there was a faster turnover, 'Not quite the turnover of today,' she suggested; 'we did get to know our patients a little more in those days.' As a sister she enjoyed the 'bustle' of surgical nursing. Liz Carter of the Royal Masonic Hospital found that the attraction of working on a surgical ward was seeing positive results. Patients would come in to have their operation, and it was then up to the nurses to keep them infection free so the patient could be nursed back to as healthy a state as possible. 'It was result oriented,' Liz added. 'Surgery I think had everything that nursing could offer. You felt you were getting real satisfaction.'

When she was sister of the surgical ward at the Royal Hospital, Sheffield, in the 1950s Margaret Webster found operations day very demanding on her nursing time. She had to allocate nurses to take the patients to theatre and stay with them until their return; this often meant having two nurses missing at any one time. There were no assistant nurses in those days, so the ward orderly was highly important. The orderly would take patients to the X-ray and other departments and help the nurses with heavy patients. As sister she also had to supervise the medical students who were learning how to dress wounds, shorten drainage tubes and take out sutures. She also had to teach them to provide sufficient pain-killers to enable her patients to be pain-free. On the private wards the allocation of nurses to theatre was often more of a problem. Doreen Tennant, at the Queen Elizabeth Hospital, Birmingham, could have as many as three nurses missing in theatre because of three different surgeons. Later, as a surgical ward sister, she was entirely in control of the waiting list, ensuring that no patient had to wait long.

A lot of patients had carcinoma of the bowel requiring perineal excision of the rectum [the removal of bowel and rectum], along with others who also needed major surgery. So it was not wise to have seven or eight of these patients all at the same time. The same with carcinoma of the breast; I did not want too many at any one time so I spaced them. This way we could keep a better balance and give more attention.

Margaret Webster found the same when she moved to a post as sister of the neurosurgery ward at Queen Elizabeth Hospital, Birmingham, between 1959 and 1963.

As sister, I had to review the waiting list for admission; I had a major input into who was to be admitted. I could say not only the number of patients I wanted in but the type as well. Too many of one condition would stretch my resources; the consultant knew that and left it to me. The waiting list was always in my office.

At this time any unconscious head injury patients were nursed on the neurological ward, where the nurses employed the technique of cooling, using a type of water-blanket. The patients had a permanent rectal thermometer and once the temperature was lowered the nurses would put a bed cradle and sheet over their body with a fan to keep the temperature stable. They also nursed patients with Parkinson's disease, who had a stereotactic operation (akin to microwaving the thalamus). Specifically for this operation, the very first orderly was trained to scrub up in theatre.

A constant concern to Margaret Webster was the cancellation of operations.

The consultant I worked with often used to cancel the last patient on the operating list. He knew this infuriated me because the patient was prepared and then disappointed. It was important; the patient had not eaten that day and then had to get prepared for the operation the next day. One day I'd had a rough time and the consultant and I had a bit of a bust up. This was not unusual as I had had a few with him. Following this he said, 'Sister you can forget a present from me this year.' And I did not get one. Most years we did extremely well, but not that year. He stuck to his guns and I stuck to mine. We soon sorted it out of course.

The other hectic time on surgical wards was theatre list day, a very busy time. Nil by mouth was the order of the day. Any nurse who has ever given a drink or breakfast to a patient on the morning theatre list will remember the reaction. 'I did that,' said Janet Bailey.

We had had a dreadful night. There were two patients with the same surname and I hardly need to tell you that in the early morning rush, I got them mixed up. My, did I get it in the neck. Sister was right, it was inexcusable. If it had been an important medication I would have taken greater care.

Joan Pease was sister of a very busy male surgical ward at Nottingham General Hospital from 1951 to 1953. She found it very rewarding but very hard work, particularly when they were 'on take'.

On take, meant that my ward would take all the emergency surgeries for a particular period of time. In the time that we were on take we had to shift out our patients who were fit enough to other wards or annexes. The patients we received in were all the big surgery of that week. Then we would be faced with the job of sorting priorities out, not only the new patients but also the ones that had been moved. It was a hectic time.

Joan found that sisters of the other wards would soon be on to her, especially if she was taking too long to get 'her' patients out of 'their' wards.

Surgical nursing could be quite alarming at times. Audrey Philips found this out more than once. One sister would have the surgical patients outside on the veranda at St Thomas's Hospital. Fresh air, she said, was good for recovery. One night there was a tremendous thunderstorm and the nurses had to get the thirty-two patients back in on their metal beds. 'I was not the only nurse who was terrified,' she said. 'I have always been frightened of storms; there were these dreadful flashes of lightning and loud claps and crashes of thunder. Fortunately the patients were all male; they found the whole thing very amusing.' On another occasion she had a patient whose operation wound burst. In training she had been taught to cover burst wounds with a pad of sterile gauze soaked in warm saline, to avoid the patient going into shock. Confronted with the real thing for the first time she just covered the wound with something, but it certainly was not sterile gauze soaked in warm saline. Calling for assistance she suddenly realized what she had done. She told the sister, who reassured her that all would be well. Nevertheless she still expected the patient to go into shock, she also worried that she might have introduced infection. However, he survived.

Surgery could be stressful. Margaret Watts trained at Farnborough Hospital, and for the practical part of her final examination in 1945 there was a ten-minute viva in front of a physician and a surgeon. The surgeon asked her what she would do about a patient who had had a thyroidectomy within the last twenty-four hours and was now showing signs of distressed breathing. She answered that beside the bed when a patient came back to the ward from theatre they always had a sterile tray with some stitch cutters or a clip remover. Nurses would observe the patient for signs of respiratory distress as there could be bleeding if a ligature slipped when the blood pressure rose on consciousness; the resultant haemorrhaging could press on the trachea and inhibit breathing. When this occurred it was important for the nurse to open the wound to relieve the pressure. For an inexperienced nurse even the thought of this procedure was frightening.

When she was the sister of the surgical ward at the Royal Free Hospital, Joan Page arrived on duty in the morning to see a woman who had had a partial thyroidectomy sitting up in bed breathing with considerable difficulty.

Stood by her bed was a frightened night staff nurse who had asked for but had not got help from the night sister, I knew the nurse and she already guessed what I would do. She had sensibly prepared a tray for the removal of clips. I went to wash my hands while instructing a nurse to phone the houseman and tell theatre to prepare for an emergency. I then evacuated a huge haematoma, allowing the lady to breathe more easily, and gave morphine. The houseman arrived and phoned the consultant who immediately came to the ward and said to him, 'How dare you allow my patients to haemorrhage!' I at once interrupted and explained what had happened; the consultant knew she could leave it to me to see the night sister. I certainly did!

Earlier, as head nurse on night duty, Joan arrived on the surgical ward at Guy's Hospital to find total silence. Every patient and nurse looked very strained, and sister had a face like thunder. Joan said, 'Oh sister, what ever is the matter?' She looked up for a moment, and then all the frustration of the day poured out. 'I have had a dreadful day,' she said. She recited some of the day's irritations, ending with, 'and that stupid new junior boiled up the colostomy bag in the new milk saucepan – the new milk saucepan would you believe!' The thought of this was too much for Joan so she replied, with a slight smile, 'How awful, just give me the report and then I'll make you a cup of Horlicks!' Fortunately, after a moment's thought sister saw the funny side of the situation and laughed, then the whole ward relaxed.

Surgical nursing was always heavy work with few lifting aids. Helen Baig (née Souster) began her nursing career on the eye and ear surgical ward in 1941 at Bradford Royal Infirmary. At sixteen and a half years old she was not deemed strong enough for the heavy lifting involved in nursing. At that time, following an operation for cataracts, patients came back to the ward with pads on both eyes and a Buller shield (a metal covering that went over the eye-pad dressings to prevent accidental rubbing of the eye) over the top. The patients were not allowed to move at all, so they were nursed flat on their backs for at least a week. At all times they had to be lifted on and off bedpans, lifted not rolled to change sheets and lifted to be fed; they were mostly elderly, so they were often very heavy. The relief for the patient came when one eye pad was removed after a week and then they were allowed one pillow. There was no such relief for the nurses; sister was not having passengers on her ward, however young or small, and Helen had to join in the lifting with the rest of the nurses.

On the surgical ward where Sylvia Kemp worked, the sister had a unique method of signalling for what she wanted. When she wanted a per rectum tray she would put her hand out from behind the screen with her finger pointed in the air. When she wanted a sphygmomanometer an arm would appear with her hand grasping it just above the elbow. She would not check whether anyone had seen these signals; she just knew someone had. Before any wound dressings were done, this same sister would also call the nurse into the office and ask her about cross-infection and the names of infections that could enter a wound.

111

Barbara Hare also found that she had to be on her toes when she was on the surgical ward. Sister Johnson, on male surgical, will for ever live in her memory, for she had the disconcerting habit of saying to junior nurses, 'Mr Jones in bed number three, how is he sitting, how is he doing at the moment, what is the level of his intravenous drip?'

> We had to know this at any time of the day so on this ward we quickly learned the power of observation. We had to, sister would go mad if you did not know. After forty years of nursing, observation is still an integral part of my life. I know I still take note of day-to-day events without actually being consciously aware of it. Sister Johnson drummed it in to us, for that I will be eternally grateful.

During the Second World War, Joan Eddings and many other nurses were moved from Westminster Hospital, London, where she was in training, to Park Prewett Hospital, Basingstoke. Park Prewett was a large mental hospital that had been turned into an emergency facility ready to receive wounded servicemen. The wards were huge, with fifty or sixty beds soon to be filled with servicemen. There was little basic equipment.

> The shock of the move from a teaching hospital to this old-fashioned hospital was great. Sister had us cleaning and polishing, there seemed to be copper and brass everywhere. Linen was boiled or steamed in a small, primitive autoclave. Fiercely proud, sister set about bringing it up to Westminster Hospital standards. She also ensured that discipline for us was just as strict.

There were no sterilizing packs so the nurses had to make their own. Sterilization of instruments on the ward was done on small paraffin stoves. To keep these clean the nurses had to carry their own pricker (a thin piece of wire). The flame on a paraffin heater came out of a little hole which had to be kept dirt free with the pricker. Nevertheless to Joan Eddings it proved to be the most interesting time in her nursing, particularly when she was allocated to work on

112

the facio-maxillary ward. On this ward young servicemen came in with terrible burns and injuries and practically had to have their faces rebuilt. Sir Harold Gillis was the surgeon in charge, she remembers. 'It was a wonderful team to work with. We were up against infections and in a moment germs could destroy months of work.'

Throughout the war years soap was desperately scarce in hospitals. The Queen Elizabeth Hospital, Birmingham, was in a crisis and advertised in the local paper. Doreen Tennant remembers that they were inundated with soap from people who must have been giving some of their own meagre rations.

I was sent by sister to collect some of this soap. We had to go to a porter called Feddy Brown and he opened a door to an Aladdin's cave of soap. Soap was piled to the ceiling, I can still remember the smell – it was wonderful, Yardley, Coty, Lifebuoy. It was a joy to us and certainly the patients.

During her nurse training at the Radcliffe Hospital, Oxford, Betty Blacklaw was one of the first nurses to have penicillin in 1944. It was first discovered as a mould in 1929 by Sir Alexander Fleming but was not widely used as an antibiotic until the middle of the Second World War, and even then was reserved almost exclusively for injured servicemen. Two wards at Radcliffe Hospital had been given over to the Australian Sir Howard W. Florey and the German Dr Ernst B. Chain. These two were instrumental in isolating and purifying the active ingredients of penicillin and later introducing it to patients. Betty Backlaw had suffered severe sinusitis and this required an operation to relieve the symptoms. Post-operatively she suffered severe infection. She was introduced to the wonders of penicillin and the pain of its administration. It was administered by slow intramuscular drip at three drops a minute, and she felt every drop day and night. A large needle was used, which kept coming out, adding to the discomfort. She was nursed by her friend Bella Blandford (née Keech), also a nurse in training. During the night the pain was so bad she used to plead with Bella to remove the needle.

Bella also became a patient when she had to have her tonsils removed. The consultant, Mr Macbeth, did not take them out under general anaesthetic; as she was a nurse he used a local. The anaesthetist administered this while she sat in a chair, and the consultant dissected them; he would have either used the guillotine or the snare method of removal. She remembers, 'It was great for a while, that was until the anaesthetic wore off, then I was in great pain, but I was pleased that I did not get an infection and have to go through the discomfort Betty had suffered.'

On the surgical ward where Bella worked there were thirty breakfasts to prepare. Since it was war time, eggs were scarce, but relatives sometimes brought them for the patients.

Each morning we would collect the eggs; their name had usually been put on by the relatives or we put them on. The relatives often gave different cooking instructions, and off we would go to the kitchen to cook them. The name invariably came off while they were boiling and I can't tell you the amount of arguing that went on because it was not 'their' egg that you had given them.

Patients' recovery following the administration of penicillin amazed everyone involved. Shocked at the multiple injuries soldiers were admitted with, the nurses were equally shocked at the remarkable recoveries due to its use. Margaret Ollerton vividly remembers the first use of penicillin in liquid form at Manchester Royal Hospital. She was directed by the sister to be in charge of a soldier with gas gangrene wounds in both his arms and legs; the wounds smelled foul and he was not expected to survive. To her delight he started to rally. 'To see these wounds begin to show signs of healing due to the administration of penicillin was one of the most extraordinary events in my nursing career. The soldier made a full recovery.' Another patient on the ward had been a sailor on a minesweeper. He suffered from amoebic dysentery and liver abscesses that needed draining, and was very ill. Margaret said, 'He did not sleep during the night and used to talk to me endlessly about his adventures in the North Atlantic where he helped rescue other seamen. He impressed me so much I married him, temporarily ending my nursing career of course.'

Avril Vincent (née Williamson) trained at the London Hospital and was placed on what she had been led to believe was the surgical ward with the most fearsome sister. On her first day the sister personally took her on the wound-dressing round. She took her to every patient, painstakingly showing her how to do the dressing, and how to probe a wound to prevent it healing from the outside in. The next day she designated her to do the dressing round on her own. 'Sister trusted us to do it properly,' Avril said. 'I am glad she did. Shortly after this, all the patients were moved because a contingent of sailors who had been torpedoed was to be admitted.' They had been swimming in a sea of burning oil, so they were severely burnt in the upper chest, arms and face. They came from Tilbury Docks, having had some initial first aid.

We cleaned them up as best we could but it was painful, painstaking work; many were terrified of the possibility of facial disfigurement. We were using tulle-gras over the wounds, a gauze impregnated with petroleum jelly, and Milton in an 'onion salad bag'; it was like a plastic envelope over the burnt area. The Milton would drip in the bag at one end and drain from the other, keeping the wound clean. Some of the poor men were enveloped in bandages and sister would send to the nurses' home for cigarette holders for these patients, as this was the only way they could safely smoke.

The surgical implantation of a tissue or organ is a relatively modern development. With the careful matching of the donor's and recipient's tissues, together with the use of drugs that suppress the recipient's immune response, great advances have been made since the first heart transplant in 1967. Now it is commonplace to transplant kidneys, lungs, livers, pancreases and other organs. In 1985 Brenda Beech was working as a sister in an eye clinic at a general hospital. It had been the practice that medical staff removed eyes from donated bodies for transplantation. She was approached and encouraged to attend an eye retrieval course at the UK transplant centre in Bristol. With some trepidation she agreed. The technique entailed the removal of the cornea not the vitreous. A few sleepless nights later and having moved from practice to the removal from cadavers she returned to her hospital. She was never very enthusiastic about this job but on learning that one of the first sets of corneas

115

she had removed had been successfully used in Birmingham after a major accident she felt it was all worthwhile.

Admissions day on a surgical ward could be a very busy time. Shortly after her promotion to sister, Sylvia Kemp was anxious to impress. With the list of new admissions she was at the ward entrance waiting to welcome the patients and direct them to their beds. She was also expecting a new consultant to visit the ward.

> This young man came to the office door. He was almost a boy to me; I asked him his name and could not find it on the list. I told him to wait and went to check again. While on the phone suddenly the penny dropped, and when it did I was highly embarrassed. I went to him and said, 'You are not J.M. Kelly, the new consultant, are you?' What a start! After that he always referred to me as the sister who tried to get him into bed on our first meeting.

When Joan Jenkins was nursing at St George's Hospital in 1936, seven young Royal Air Force men were admitted. They were visiting London and standing at the railings of Buckingham Palace. A car careered off the road and drove into them. All were badly injured, and six died on the ward. She recalls, 'I was with one of these young men when he died, it was so terribly tragic.' The one survivor had to have surgery to amputate both legs; she was assigned his care. Most remarkably in the same ward was the driver of the car.

> We were told, but did not need to be told, that we must never let anything out about what had happened. Every day an equerry came up from the palace with whatever the RAF man needed. Before I left St Georges I had the pleasure of seeing this man on his 'tin legs' as he called them.' He was transferred to Carshalton to be fitted with the legs and trained to use them. When he had learned to fully cope with them he returned to the hospital to proudly show us his new walking abilities.

Doreen Tennant started nurse training in September 1944, when the surgical wards at Queen Elizabeth Hospital, Birmingham, were still swamped with D-Day patients. The convoys would usually arrive at night and officers would initially be sorted from other ranks. Then came the job of sorting out the physical priorities. Placed on a ward for officers she had no idea what had happened with most of them, other than they were severely burned and had limbs missing. Most were apparently blast and burn injuries in the tank regiments. The ward had previously held thirty beds with one large room and four smaller ones. The army had brought in small 2 feet 6 inch beds so that more people could be accommodated.

There were beds everywhere. I came on duty at 7.00 a.m. and went into a room and one of the soldiers called out, in a broad Scottish voice, 'I need some newspaper, I must have some newspaper, nurse!' Paper was very scarce, with most newspapers reduced to one or two sheets. I went to Sister and she encouraged me to find some paper. We managed to collect enough to satisfy him. 'He said, 'Spread it round the floor,' which we did. 'Now open my bag.' It seemed he was used to giving orders. In the bag was his kilt, he was in the 51st Highland Division. When the kilt was spread over the newspaper we could see him visibly relax.

This same sister picked up from the padre that one of the soldiers who was very ill and not expected to live wanted to see a newborn baby; he said he did not know what a newborn baby looked like. Two of us were detailed to push his bed, with the padre leading, along the corridor into the lift and up two floor levels. When we got there the maternity sister had been alerted and produced two new babies for the soldier to see and hold. It was such an emotional experience for him and us, we all ended in tears.

9 Theatre Sisters

It was not continuous drama in theatre, I could not have coped
with that. Exciting at times, it was not always the stuff of television.

Margaret Marsh, theatre sister,
Harrogate General Hospital, 1956

Before the end of the nineteenth century an operating theatre was far
removed from the high-tech pristine environment we know today. An
open coal fire warmed the room; this fire would also be used for
heating water. In earlier days the room would sometimes double as
the ward kitchen. The main lighting came from large uncurtained
windows. During the operation, the table was protected with a
rubber sheet, and there was a large tray of sawdust on the floor to
catch blood. The operating table would be washed down and a fresh
blanket and pillow placed on it between each operation. The surgeon
and his assistants often operated in their outdoor suits without gloves
or masks, and usually without protective clothing. If a white coat was
worn, it would rarely be washed and its blood-stained appearance
would be proudly displayed. At any one operation only eight rock
sponges were allowed for each patient. These would be washed, and
following the introduction of Lister's aseptic principles of 1865
dipped in carbolic and dried ready for another patient.

The first operating theatre sisters were appointed in the early
1860s, their theatre duties secondary to those of their ward. In the
theatre they were responsible for the cleanliness and good order of
equipment and for making it ready for operations. They did not have
any other nursing assistance, apart from a nurse who accompanied
the patient and stayed throughout the operation. By the1880s the

rules began to change. This was almost entirely due to sisters being appointed to surgical wards; it was now this sister who attended in the theatre throughout all operations. This meant that the sister was away from her ward for long periods, but common sense soon prevailed and the decision was overturned. In many hospitals, and for many years, the theatre sister was responsible for the purchase of almost everything that was required for both theatre and the wards.

Dr Laurence Humphrey, in his *Manual for Nurses*, explained the duties of a theatre sister in 1891. Often single-handed, the theatre sister was instructed to be attentive, on the lookout and ready with anything that might possibly be required by the surgeon. It might simply be attending to sponges – having a clean one always ready to hand and a bowl for the soiled ones. Each sponge was to be washed in warm carbolic solution and well rung out before being handed back to the surgeon, otherwise the wound would fill with water. Any other equipment and dressings that might be required by the surgeon were to be at hand ready. A bowl was also to be available if the patient was sick on recovering from the anaesthetic; with gases such as ether, nitrous oxide and chloroform, they often were. Anaesthesia was introduced in the 1840s, commonly used by the 1860s and used at all operations by the 1890s; this allowed for the first successful appendectomy to be performed in 1887.

Before any dressing was applied the nurse had again to be prepared with a clean warm carbolic solution and a fresh sponge to wipe away the blood and clean the surrounding parts which had been soiled. So as not to pull at the sutures – although it maximized the potential for infection – the nurse was directed that in sponging, movement should be towards the wound, not away from it. The wound was then covered. It was not the most sterile of procedures, hand scrubbing was not considered important and certainly it was many years before hand scrubbing was only considered complete after three minutes.

In the days before improved anaesthetics and life-support systems operating theatres were places of acute tension, with operations conducted under constant time constraints. Before anaesthetics were in wide use surgery was about both skill and speed. Operating theatres have therefore always been places for high drama, with times of furious activity and total concentration. But as Margaret Marsh, who trained at King's College Hospital and worked at Harrogate General Hospital pointed out, the personality of the theatre sister was important in the efficient running and management of theatre. Surgeons could be arrogant and deliberately difficult at times. Even the anaesthetists could have their moments under periods of tension. It was not unusual to have instruments and swabs thrown around the theatre, accompanied by a great deal of swearing. The sister had to know their various foibles and characteristics and manage them accordingly.

Jane Carter was in theatre when a new surgeon from one of the London hospitals threw an instrument across the floor. Sister calmly said, 'We do not do that sort of thing in this theatre.' In the main the surgeon would usually thank the theatre team for a job well done at the end of a particularly difficult operation and at the end of the day.

It seems that nurses either loved or hated operating theatre work. Opinions ranged from extremely boring, with the patients unconscious all the time, to challenging and exciting, depending on the nature of the surgery and the staff involved. Margaret Marsh loved her time as theatre sister; she felt she was working with a well-defined and cohesive team. She found it was up to her to develop a smooth-running system. The staff, she felt, 'had to be trustworthy team players. Nobody saw if they dropped something or made a mistake, so they had to be trustworthy. Once you got a good team you just had to keep an eye on things; they would ensure the instrument sets were put together properly and any extras as needed.'

Love it or hate it, an operating theatre had to be kept clean. Saturdays were usually the cleaning days. The sister would have ensured that the junior nurse collected all the enamel bowls, jugs, basins, porringers, kidney dishes, plus her coffee jugs, and took them to the big sink. With a large scrubbing brush and scouring powder, she set to work. Another nurse would clean the anaesthetic trolley along with the rubber tubing and mouthpieces, with hot water and antiseptic. All needles were sharpened on a carbon block and sister would rub the point against a piece of cotton wool; if the wool stuck it meant there was a hooked end and so it was sharpened again. As well as the instruments there would be the preparation of needles threaded with catgut, and purse-string sutures and carbolic swabs made ready. The nurse would also be expected to have checked the first batch of swabs and instruments ready for the sister to double-check. The making up of supplies of sterile water, saline and boracic solution was also done at this time. All instruments and syringes would be washed, counted, cleaned and oiled, then set up in packs and sterilized in the theatre ready for use. In the more relaxed times of general cleaning, Reg Commander became acquainted with Felix Mendelssohn's Italian Symphony, courtesy of Sister Theatre.

Until the introduction of a central sterile supplies department (CSSD) in the 1960s nurses made up all the dressings from abdominal ones to the small swabs they wrapped on forceps. These were sometimes stapled with wire clips, so that they would show up on X-ray. Many surgeons became impatient during a swab count and would often just go ahead and close the wound, so this was a great advantage. Other swabs were sorted into packs of five or ten and tied with tape, always checked and counted by the sister. Most of these did not have staples so the swab count was always of the highest importance. After any operation the swabs would be recounted and if the count had been wrong in the first place it would cause delays. Any junior nurse will remember being the 'dirty nurse' hovering around the operation table picking up messy swabs and placing them in rows of six or ten on a rubber mat or hanging them on a swab rack. They will also remember the accusing eyes when the sister found they were one swab short, only to recheck and find two swabs stuck together. The same applied to surgical instruments: clamps, forceps, scissors, scalpels, all were fastidiously counted.

Margaret Sheehan thoroughly enjoyed her role as theatre sister at the Salford Royal Hospital. Trained long before central sterile supply systems and theatre technicians, she recalls nurses being responsible for all the equipment in the theatre. They checked and replaced gas cylinders on the Boyle's anaesthetic trolleys. Rubber tubing and mouthpieces were placed in a bucket of boiling water liberally laced with Dettol. Prior to an operation the nurse chose the necessary instruments for each case and boiled them in a sterilizer adjacent to the theatre. China trays were filled with a solution of Lysol for the sterilization of needles, scissors and scalpels. Any visitors to the theatre were watched with an eagle eye to ensure that there was no danger of contamination. As theatre sister Margaret was on call twenty-four hours a day and was often called out at night and escorted by a porter to the hospital from the sisters' home.

Earlier in her career Audrey Phillips was appointed to take charge of the emergency theatre at St Thomas's Hospital. It was situated on the basement floor along with the pipes and other paraphernalia. With another nurse she worked thirty nights on and then had a week off. She had been told there would not be too much extra work.

> This was not quite true. Night after night there would be seven or eight operations, duodenal ulcers, partial gastrectomies, oesophagectomies, bronchostomies and fractures; we were busy right through the night. The day staff would come on and be most unhappy as they thought we should have had time to do other work.

When Audrey had gained greater experience she was earmarked to work with the more difficult surgeons; she would not stand any nonsense. 'You talk about throwing a pair of forceps on the floor, I have seen trays dumped on the floor. Swab counts were often difficult times; if you were unsure about a count you had to stand your ground until you were sure.'

At Wolverhampton Royal Hospital, Reg Commander (later the Revd Commander) found that when working in theatre he would also be called to the wards to prepare the patients for theatre. If the operation site needed shaving, Harry Blower, the hospital barber, did it, but if he was not there it was the job of the male nurse. Reg remembers using an open razor. 'Without any training I set to. If I nicked the patient I ran the risk of remarks from the surgeon like, "Ah, I see you've started the operation, would you like to carry on, Commander?" The patient would be rushed back to the ward deeply unconscious with an airway *in situ*, leaving the recovery responsibilities with the ward staff.

Reg was regularly given the opportunity to scrub up.

> 'Hutch' the surgeon would encourage me with remarks like, 'Take your fingers out, sonny, and move over.' Most surgeons would seal off 'bleeders' by diathermy, but Hutch would have none of it. All his patients had to be clipped and tied off with catgut. This was particularly difficult with a mastectomy. We

could have as many as two dozen Spencer-Wells forceps in use at a time.

For each operation instruments, fresh bowls, disinfectant, gowns and gloves were made ready. There was great excitement – and dread – when a nurse was asked to scrub up, gown up and retract. This meant holding some organ or other out of the way with a retractor. Sisters could be more closely involved with the operation, holding retractors and Spencer-Wells forceps while bleeding points were ligatured, snipping the catgut ends, passing the appropriate instruments, keeping her eye on the suction machine and producing the correct needle and catgut to order, at the same time staying calm and in control. The dread for any junior nurse was being asked questions. The language of theatre was different from ward language, with a diploma in zoology often more appropriate than one in biology. However, Margaret felt that the most important nurse during an operation was not the sister or the scrubbed nurse – anyone could be taught to scrub, she argued. It was the nurse who was serving the scrubbed nurse, who was watching and anticipating what she wanted – the runner. If more swabs or instruments were needed she was expected to anticipate this need. Margaret also thought the most important role for theatre sister was teaching.

When Sylvia Kemp was training in theatre, the sister would have instrument classes every week for the junior nurses. They had to know by heart the general set and the extras that individual surgeons liked – surgeons' extras. When they were new to theatre nurses were not allowed to scrub for operations, but they would act as runner. The runner's job was a huge, uncompromising test of instrument classes. Usually in a hurry she had to be able to identify any instrument sister or the surgeon required. Sylvia's sister had a unique system for helping new nurses to remember. At her instruction lesson she would say, 'National problem'. The class would puzzle over this and then someone would come up with, 'Parking a car', which would provoke a scramble and a nurse would find a Parker Carr clamp. Then she would put her hand over her eye and someone would produce a Nelson's clamp. A smoking action brought a Dunhill's. One male nurse was asked to produce a gynaecology instrument. 'Liquorice allsorts, liquorice allsorts,' she repeated. He said 'Bassett's' and she responded irritably, 'Wilkinson's' and someone produced the appropriate cannula. 'She would have done better saying razor blades!' he grumbled.

Billie Cullen was a sister at the Radcliffe Hospital, Oxford. Being near Brize Norton airfield they received many soldiers from the Second World War Normandy landings. The injured servicemen would arrive in the afternoon and a list would be made up for that evening's operating theatre. Working on night duty on one wing of the hospital she would be called on to open the theatre ready for operations.

It was so very sad seeing these young men with gunshot wounds and the most appalling multiple fractures. It was the bayonet wounds that got to us; we could hardly imagine the brutal fighting they had been through. Rather than treat the fractures in France they would be put in splints and plaster and these would be removed in theatre to uncover some frightful sights. Thank goodness the patient was unconscious and did not have to see the looks on our faces. Then in the bustle of theatre we just got on with it of course.

The team would already have been informed as to whether it would be an amputation or repair. To cope with the demand two extra operating tables were introduced so the nurses would be setting up sets for each table. As she pointed out, 'This was on top of the day list, but it all worked very well.'

New nurses could be the bane of a sister's life. The great day came for Margaret Ollerton (née Woodington) at Manchester Royal Infirmary when she was to scrub up for the first time for a lumbar sympathectomy. Some of the instruments were sterilized in Lysol, and they had to be taken out and washed in sterile water. The patient was already on the table anaesthetized. But as Margaret said, 'I had only been used to working in theatre as the un-scrubbed nurse, consequently the worst happened, I forgot to put on my sterile gloves and contaminated the lot.' She was spotted by the theatre sister and the operation was immediately abandoned. Margaret was expecting a severe telling-off from the sister, but the surgeon calmly interceded and said, 'That's a blessing, I can now go and see my husband off.'

124

He was an officer in the army and off she went!

The trials of being new to theatre work also fell on David Rogers at Sheffield Royal Infirmary. He had been in the theatre only a few days when the surgeon looked directly at him and told him to readjust the theatre light; working on a mandible resection of the jaw he wanted to change his angle of sight. Not ever having touched the light let alone adjusted it, David started to pull and twist it, and ended up with the light shining on the patient's lower abdomen. Very patiently the surgeon suggested that if he was going to leave it there, he could always remove the patient's appendix instead.

Ann Grose (née Chick) was a junior staff nurse and was preparing the sterile trays in the theatre for an operation. The final job was to lay up the bowl trolley. To do this a nurse would put a sterilized cloth over the top of the trolley and place a suitable bowl in the hole in the centre. Unfortunately the bowl she chose was too small. When she started to pour in the hot water it fell through the hole, making an awful clatter and spilling water everywhere. Ordered out of the theatre by the theatre sister she stood outside the door wondering what to do. Some time later the sister came for her and took her back; she was by now surprisingly pleasant.

On theatre days the nurses and surgeons continued until the last person on the list was operated on; there was no question of putting patients off because time was running out. At the end of the list, when the last patient had been returned to the wards and the surgeons and anaesthetists had left, it was clean-up time again. The staff would have to make the theatre ready for the next day. The floors were again scrubbed, either by the orderly if they were lucky enough to have one or by nursing staff, using buckets of hot water and Lysol. The strong smell of Lysol added to the smell of ether was the unique hospital smell, and was remembered by all who experienced it. They were the smells that got into the back of people's throats and the public always associated them with a hospital visit.

Working in theatre could entail taking on different tasks. Olga Marshall was detailed by the sister at Manchester Royal Infirmary to help out in the dental department. Here there was a very small sterilizer for instruments, which had to be kept on the boil. A man with both legs amputated was brought in strapped in a wheelchair. The porter and Olga transferred him to the dental chair. There were no straps on this chair, so it was Olga's job to hold him there while he was anaesthetized. As she explained: 'The extraction took a long time, far too long! Although I had filled the sterilizer with water it was boiling away. To my horror the metal started to buckle and then melt. I could not believe my eyes, especially when the metal started to run down the wall tiles.' Caught between either ignoring it or letting the anaesthetized patient go she chose to ignore it. The dentist was no help at all; he had his job to do, and he also suffered from a lack of a sense of humour. Of course she had to report the incident to the theatre sister, who also suffered a lack of humour. 'Oh my, what a dressing-down I got!'

Hardly able to draw breath from receiving her final results on a Saturday morning Audrey Jones commenced in theatre at St Nicholas Hospital in Plumstead on the Sunday. The sister was off for the weekend and she found herself in charge. As luck would have it there was an emergency. She had to prepare the theatre, then scrub up.

> I was given a hell of a time during the operation; the surgeon had some sort of a personality change, he was awful. When you had to act as assistant to the surgeon, it made no difference if you were an experienced sister or a junior staff nurse. He did have the grace to apologize later, but it did shake my confidence for a little while.

Undoubtedly the worst job for a new nurse in theatre was watching the removal of amputated limbs. One student nurse was a little too near the operating table and was told to hold a leg while it was being amputated above the knee. Unfortunately, when it was amputated she was not told what to do with it. On her own initiative, therefore, she carefully stood it in one of the floor bowls and commenced to wheel it out of the theatre, quite unaware that the surgical team had stopped to watch what she was doing. Carefully holding the leg upright she wheeled it through the theatre doors and into the instrument room. 'Well,' said the surgeon, 'now she has legged it we will carry on!' Theatre was often the place for this sort of 'gallows' humour.

Used to seeing adult patients in the operating theatre Helen Baig at the Bradford Royal Infirmary found the procession of children on

126

the French Red Cross; they were successful in setting up their Women's Hospital Corps and establishing hospitals in Paris and Wimereux, near Boulogne. Eventually the War Office gave permission for them to found the Women's Military Hospital in Endell Street, London.

Midwifery is as old as humanity; women have been acting as midwives since long before it was chronicled in historical records. Its origins are vague, but it was natural for women who had experienced a birth of their own to assist new mothers at their births. From the Middle Ages onwards nursing has been dogged by stories of unscrupulous midwives, but there were also many respectable and capable women who attended at childbirth. Throughout those years, of course, the birth took place in the home, there were no hospitals or other institutions for expectant mothers.

The first schools for midwives were opened in the nineteenth century; here they were given twice-weekly lectures. The first maternity hospital, the Queen Charlotte Maternity Hospital, London, opened later that century. Also in London, the Ladies' Obstetric College, founded in 1864, accommodated the daughters of professional men, who attended lectures and became midwives. So for the women who could afford them, trained private nurses were available. But, as always, this service was denied to the poor, who had to rely on midwives who might have had some instruction but who mostly picked up their trade as they went along.

In 1867, Florence Nightingale organized a training school for midwives at King's College Hospital, London. Unfortunately there was a severe outbreak of infection (puerperal sepsis), and as a consequence the project was abandoned. Learning from this experience, Nightingale showed characteristic foresight by suggesting that separate rooms be used to limit infection and reduce the unacceptable mortality rate. She proposed an institution for the training of midwives and maternity nurses in her book *Introductory Notes on Laying-in Hospitals*, published in 1871. In the following year, the Obstetric Society of London established an examination for midwives in response to their findings that untrained women were widely practising midwifery.

Although it was seen as a lucrative branch of nursing, the old style

tonsil and adenoid days very upsetting. There would be about thirty of them twice a week at the end of the adult list. Very frightened, these tots in their little rubber caps and capes would be led by a nurse into the anaesthetic room. They were given chloroform and then carried to the operating table. Their tonsils were taken out with a guillotine, and a cotton swab wrapped on forceps was held into each cavity. The children were then placed on their sides while their adenoids were scraped out into a metal container fastened on the side of the table, where the tonsils had already gone. The children were then taken back to the ward, where they were put top to tail in a bed. 'It was a gory business,' Helen remembers. 'At the end of the list the theatre staff had to pour the contents of the container through a big colander and send what remained to the boiler room for incineration.'

Margaret Watts spent only a short time as a staff nurse before being promoted to sister. Following her Part 1 midwifery, which had been increased from six to nine months after the end of the Second World War to keep as many nurses in midwifery as possible because of an expected baby boom, she took charge of theatre as a temporary sister at Farnborough Hospital. As preparation she was given a short introduction to theatre work at the Royal London Ear, Nose and Throat Hospital. After four months the matron offered her the permanent post. Margaret accepted and to start with her office was a padded cell. The huts that the theatre occupied had obviously been used before the war as a psychiatric unit and this was the only place for an office. She found it quite amusing inviting the medical staff in there for a cup of tea.

In this post she was involved with what was possibly the first use of curare in the UK. Obtained from certain tropical trees, it acted on the central nervous system, causing temporary paralysis of the diaphragm. One of the anaesthetists had researched its use as a relaxant and wanted to try it. The anaesthetist had to sign a declaration that he was taking full responsibility, along with another colleague. 'It was quite a dramatic moment really,' said Margaret, 'with the four of us standing there and the patient on artificial ventilation. The patient recovered without any problems.'

Madeline Clifford's first experience in the operating theatre was at Knowle Hospital, Fareham, in 1950. A mental hospital, it had a theatre for minor operations. Up to the 1960s most mental hospitals had their own operating and dental theatres, and pathology and X-ray departments. A doctor would travel regularly from London with his own theatre sister to perform any operations. A local anaesthetist would also attend. Prefrontal leucotomy was the principal operation of the time. The theatre sister was clearly in charge throughout the operations, ensuring that everything was prepared and sterilized. The patient, who had been made ready by shaving the front part of the head, was put under a general anaesthetic. Then two holes were bored into the front of the skull with a trephine and parts of the nerve fibres of the brain were severed with a scalpel. The doctor often brought junior medical students with him and not surprisingly during these procedures she saw as many as two or three of these students faint.

I quite got used to this and was always ready with cups of tea. At the time this operation was considered to be very successful for treating severe compulsive behaviour problems, although in later years the casualties of prefrontal leucotomy tended to require prolonged hospital support for behaviour problems.

10   Women's Ward Sisters

They [patients] must know that she [the sister] cares for them even while she is checking them; or rather that she checks them because she cares for them.

Florence Nightingale to probationers, May 1872

Male medical staff vehemently resisted the idea of women-only hospitals in the nineteenth century. Their main objection was to the possibility of women being registered as doctors. Registering as a trainee nurse at Middlesex Hospital, Elizabeth Garrett Anderson went to the classes intended for medical students. She quickly outshone her classmates, so she was barred from the lecture room. In 1865 she passed the Society of Apothecaries examination and a year later established a dispensary for women in London, where thousands of poor women and children benefited, and a year later she was made a visiting physician at a children's hospital in East London. But it was 1879 before an Act was passed allowing women to enter all the medical professions. The hospital named after her became a blueprint; it was entirely staffed by women keen to nurse women and for women to study medicine. From this beginning women-only hospitals started to open in major cities throughout the country. Elizabeth Garrett Anderson was also noted for being the Mayor of Aldeburgh – she was the first female mayor in England. She died in 1917.

At the outbreak of the First World War, her daughter Dr Louisa Garrett Anderson, with Dr Flora Murray, wanted to establish a Women's Hospital Corps, but the War Office refused to countenance using the services of these two women surgeons. However, their medical expertise was welcomed in France, where they worked with

of monthly nursing, when a nurse would be employed by the more affluent for the first month following a birth, had virtually died out by the end of the nineteenth century. Nurses were being encouraged to train and were first given a one-year course in a general hospital followed by three to six months in a laying-in hospital. Laying-in hospitals were the only places that accepted in-patient maternity cases but they were always plagued by puerperal infections, with consequently high death rates. They received mothers who were so poor they could not be cared for at home, but patients were still expected to supply their own bed linen, utensils and drugs. The nurses at these hospitals were encouraged to take a diploma with the London Obstetric Society and go on to become certified midwives. There were laying-in and maternity hospitals in Ireland (Dublin and Belfast), Scotland (Glasgow and Edinburgh) and England (Manchester, Liverpool and London), which all accepted pupils for midwifery training, each of whom paid approximately 7 guineas.

At the end of the nineteenth century antenatal care was practically non-existent, and a combination of ignorance in the community and indifference from the medical authorities meant that there were far more untimely miscarriages and deaths of mothers among the poor than there should have been. The midwife would be called only when the baby was due, and other than delivering the babies her abilities would mainly be in dealing with obstetric tragedies such as obstructed labour, haemorrhage and sepsis. Post-natal management was bed-rest, which entailed at least three days prostrate, with no exertion or sudden movements. After this the head could be raised by one pillow and the patient propped up to take food. On the eighth or tenth day, if they were doing well, patients would be allowed outside the bedclothes in a dressing gown, and after a day or two more they could sit out in a chair. In delicate people this recovery time was greatly extended. There was little likelihood of a doctor attending following the birth, and little or no obstetric care. Sadly the death rate continued to remain high.

In the late 1880s designated obstetric departments were established, with the Bristol General Hospital opening one in 1887. It was concerned only with outpatients initially and there was no designated nurse to assist. It was 1892 before a nurse was detailed to attend cases in the community with a medical student. In 1894 a permanent qualified nurse was appointed. A six-bed obstetric ward was opened at the general hospital in 1896, with a nurse being sent to Queen Charlotte's Hospital, London, for training in midwifery. In 1900 Dr J.W. Ballantyne of Edinburgh University, the real pioneer of obstetric care, wrote about the frightful state of antenatal care. He also argued that a 'pre-maternal' hospital was urgently needed. He won that argument, but it was many years before midwifery won the right to have properly regulated training.

The Central Midwives' Board, which was established at the end of 1902, immediately set up a roll of midwife practitioners. This included the *bona fide* midwives who had practised for one year or more without any training. Up to this time midwifery had been to all intents and purposes uncontrolled. The Midwives Act of 1902 stated that from 1905 any woman not certified under the Act who took or used the title of midwife, would be fined £5. After 1910, no woman could attend women in childbirth, except under the direction of a qualified medical practitioner, unless certified under the Act. Any woman so doing would be liable to a fine of £10. This Act gave control of midwives to local councils, and stipulated that midwives should notify the local authority about their place of practice. The Midwife Act of 1936 provided the first state-operated service, but it was not there to provide a rounded maternity service; instead it was part of a service triad that included antenatal and post-natal provision.

More maternity hospitals were opening and providing excellent training for new midwives. In the 1930s the London Hospital trained twenty-six midwives a year. For certification, the Midwives' Board required that twenty deliveries be completed, half under instruction in hospital and the other half in the community. In the community the pupil would be taken by the district sister to one or two deliveries, then accompany a more senior pupil before attending deliveries on her own. A big shock to many nurses was the difference they found between life in the hospital and life in the community. The poverty was sometimes appalling.

Up to the First World War newborn babies both in hospital and in the community were kept in flannel binders wound round their midriffs. Mothers were also bound in abdominal binders, huckaback towelling 36 inches wide and 1¼ yards long, doubled lengthways. Its lower edge reached 4 inches below the top of the thighbone and it was bound tightly round the abdomen and fastened by 'four strong pins'; straight two-inch long pins were thought best.

Rosalie Pearce trained at the Royal Hospital, Wolverhampton, in 1913 and 1914. One of her entries in her notes from the training school covered the care of the newborn baby:

> The mother usually feeds her child for nine months, unless a further pregnancy occurs, when the child should be weaned. It is important to wean gradually, giving a feed of natural and one of artificial food alternately . . . Children should not be weaned in July, August and September as these are not the cleanest of months . . . In the dressing of the new baby it is first bound with a strip of flannel wrapped two and a half times round its body and worn continually for the first three months, after which a knitted binder could be used; second, a knitted vest; third, a napkin made of Turkish towelling; fourth, a high necked long-sleeved vest; fifth, a cotton dress, and finally a matinée coat. There was no indicator at to whether this was summer or winter attire.

Breast-feeding was almost universal and was considered the safest, the cheapest, and the best method of feed for the new baby. The great problem was the low-weight births. Up to and for some time beyond the Second World War, the outlook for premature low-birth-weight babies was gloomy. Feeding was problematic. The management of feeds was usually left to the ward sister. She was the one with the most experience at a time when little was known about substitutes for breast-feeding. She was considered the one with the expertise to decide the choice of feed, the amount and the method of feed. This was a balance between specialist nursing and common sense. There were attempts at overcoming this problem at the maternity departments of Birmingham and Bristol, where they had special premature infant departments. Expressed milk has always been recognized as a substitute for babies who cannot feed normally and it had been the practice to take this excess milk from mothers in post-natal wards. One scheme in Harrow in the 1970s was to collect excess breast milk from mothers in their own homes. As milk could be frozen the introduction of freezers made this easier.

The main textbook for midwives has been *The Textbook for Midwives* written by Margaret F. Myles. First published in 1953, this was the first textbook in which practical procedures and obstetric nursing were described in detail. Margaret Myles was the first midwife tutor appointed to the Simpson Memorial Maternity Pavilion, Edinburgh, where she taught obstetrics for fourteen years. Another much-used book for the pupil midwife was *Pictorial Midwifery* by Sir Comyns Berkeley, first published in 1926. This was fully illustrated, and was an illuminating book for young nurses who had little knowledge of such things.

The wonders of married life and even more the mystery of conception were discovered by Betty Blacklar and her student nurse colleagues at the Radcliffe Hospital, Oxford, where a family planning clinic was opened in 1946. Betty was allocated there as part of her training. Like her colleagues, she had no idea about such things; her placement did however make her popular with her friends. They would eagerly await her return to the nurses' home to get all the information they could from her. 'Looking back it was quite incongruous,' she said. 'We were there to advise on a subject that we had no experience of, let alone ever discussed.'

By the young Joan Eddings and her student colleagues at Westminster Hospital, the birth of a baby was anticipated with a mixture of curiosity and puzzlement. Working on the maternity wards the new nurses were to learn about female anatomy for the very first time. To the inexperienced girl maternity was quite an eye-opener. Having led somewhat cloistered lives, these young nurses had no idea from where the baby would appear. Sex education did not exist and parents would not discuss such things with their daughters. Sexual anatomy was not a fit topic for young girls of that day.

For Alice Carr (née Smith), her first time at a delivery was accompanied by some apprehension.

I was so unsure about what was to happen I did not realize I had my hands under the area that the baby was about to appear from until Sister said, 'You do not need to do that nurse, the babies do not drop out.' I really did expect the baby to drop out and even when she told me it wouldn't, I was still in great expectation that it would fall out and hurt itself.

A slippery challenge for a young nurse came shortly after the birth: the bathing of a newborn baby. Since many of these girls had little experience it was a very anxious time. Sue Clements, who trained at Great Ormond Street, remembers with sympathy this worrying activity. 'A very carefully laid out procedure added to the anxiety of "getting it right".' Surviving the first baby bath was like an initiation. Although there was no maternity unit at Great Ormond Street, there were plenty of opportunities for nurses to learn. Neonates with respiratory distress syndrome, cardiothoracic and neonatal problems, nephrological, gastroenterological and other abnormalities requiring specialist care were common and would be transported by ambulance within hours of birth.

Pam Grosvenor, who trained at the Western General Hospital, Edinburgh, and worked at the Princess Mary Maternity Hospital, Newcastle, thought her experience as maternity ward sister somewhat typical. 'I was a labour ward sister in a maternity unit. The ward arrangement meant that there could be several sisters on duty at the same time, although each would be in charge of her particular domain. A senior sister presided overall and was responsible for policy and management.' Whether an experienced sister or not, when it came to midwifery all were considered to be pupil midwives until training was completed. Even the night sister of the hospital rarely made a decision without calling on the maternity sister, who lived next to the ward.

As well as the routine washing of the theatre, general cleaning and other activities, night duty was spent keeping the babies quiet, as the sister of the ward slept next to the nursery. The unit was very busy, as babies did not come to order, and Pam could never quite understand why the work came in batches, so that there were hectic periods followed by comparative lulls. But the busiest period was almost always on night duty, so meals were a rarity. Apart from the routine work, the main emphasis on night duty was patient-focused, with the monitoring of the progress of labour and pain relief. Pam found that one of the most difficult judgements she had to make was when to call a doctor, especially when she knew the doctors were in desperate need of sleep themselves.

On maternity wards nurses have always had a lot of paperwork, so one time-consuming task Pam remembers well was completing all the records following a delivery. After a hectic night it was not unusual to spend one or two hours just finishing this paperwork.

Disposable nappies began to be introduced in the 1980s; prior to that, towelling, muslin and other such materials were used, which had to be boiled by the nurses. Cots were attached to the foot of the bed, with the baby almost out of the mother's reach. The babies would be brought to the mothers for breast-feeding and returned to the cots shortly after. At night they were taken to a side ward and new mothers would spend heartbreaking nights listening to them crying. One mother remembers being awake most of the night on the post-natal ward worrying about her baby while the night nurse settled down in her chair with a blanket over her and slept.

By the 1960s, following a birth, a mother would have eight to fourteen days of bed-rest. Mothers would only handle their baby for breast-feeding; otherwise the babies remained in their cots and the nurses dealt with them. Vaginal swabbing was done two or three times a day and any sutures removed after six or seven days. Breasts were checked for cracked nipples and if any mother had a lot of milk, the nurse would encourage her to express it for use in the milk kitchen for the premature babies. The babies were tightly wrapped in their clothing and then placed in their cots. Bella Blandford firmly believes the babies slept better for this. Newborn premature babies were rubbed in olive oil, wrapped in cotton wool and had little woolly hats, socks and gloves; there would also be a hot-water bottle at the top and one at the bottom of the incubator.

Brenda Beech was the sister of a premature baby unit in 1956 when a very competent and experienced midwife rushed in from a home delivery with a premature baby. Apparently she had delivered him with a pupil midwife and when they checked him, he was very small, approximately 2 pounds, and showed no sign of life. Survival rates for this weight were very low. The midwife told the pupil to wrap the baby and put it down by the side of one of the old-fashioned open-hearth ranges. After seeing to the mother, the pupil went to pick the baby up and it suddenly showed signs of life, hence the rush to the hospital. The baby survived and was discharged to his mother many weeks later; the doctor on the unit reckoned his survival was mainly due to being laid aside and unattended next to the warmth from the open hearth.

Shortly after qualifying Aileen Gardner (née Haffenden), was fortunate enough to be moved to the premature baby unit. This she found to be the most satisfying nursing she had encountered.

Everything was in miniature. The unit was not large with the incubators only taking up a small space compared to beds on a ward. The premature babies were so tiny and sadly the very early babies did not survive as they do today. I found this was the hardest to deal with in this unit.

Some specialist foods were being developed, but for the most part the feeds were prepared on the unit and carefully fed through nasal tubes. Aileen continued on the unit until she left to have a family of her own. Coincidently one of her children was premature so her baby was nursed on this same premature unit.

On one night duty on maternity Barbara Hare discovered that not all instructions from the sister could be carried out without thoroughly checking.

One night I made a big error; I was told by Sister to give a suppository to a newly admitted pregnant lady in bed four. I gave it to the lady in bed four. Unfortunately the pregnant lady who should have had it had been moved to another bed; the lady in bed four should not have had it. Sin of all sins. I lost a lot of sleep that following day.

Barbara knew that defending herself by saying she had been told to do this by sister would not be a good idea.

When Bella Blandford was at the Royal Free Hospital in the 1950s, husbands were not permitted to attend the birth. 'It was never thought of,' she said. 'Visiting was for the husband only and he was not allowed to pick up or breathe over the baby; he definitely could not sit on the bed.' As night sister at that time she would have to remove the radium needles on the gynaecology ward. Used in cancer of the uterus, fallopian tubes or vagina, they were removed and placed in a thick, heavy lead box and then taken to matron's office and deposited in the safe. Throughout this procedure an equally heavy apron had to be worn.

Ignorance of the body and women's conditions among nurses was one problem, but there was equal ignorance among younger women who became pregnant. Even the 'permissive society' of the 1960s did little to alter this situation. Young women would visit their doctor or the casualty department complaining of abdominal discomfort to be told they were pregnant. Many of them admitted that they were totally ignorant of what was happening to them. They would not even know how the baby was to be born. It was more frightening when they were admitted because of a threatened abortion; abortion is a traumatic experience for any woman, whether spontaneous or induced, and it just added to these poor girls' distress. Infections, disease, and endocrine dysfunction were among the maternal problems associated with abortion.

When new nurses had their first experience on a gynaecology ward, knowing next to nothing about bodies and especially the reproductive organs, they were often shocked at the illnesses they saw: prolapses, carcinoma of the cervix, bladder and pelvic floor abnormalities. Christine James recalls:

> I was on the gynaecology ward very early in my training. I was told by Sister to give a bedpan to one of the ladies. I still think she could have warned me because this lady had a complete prolapse of her uterus. This had to be lifted up so she could use the pan. To a young girl who had seen nothing like it before it came as quite a shock. It was really a jump into the deep end for me and my colleagues; as young girls we did not realize such things could happen to a woman's body.

Training on a gynaecology ward Wendy Carson found that the sister's standing orders were very clear: all patients were to be washed, beds made and all the usual tidying of table tops, clearing of locker tops, damp dusting, wheels pointing in the same direction, done by the stroke of 9.00 a.m. At this time the door to her office would open and she would make her grand entrance, treatment book in hand. All staff had to be inconspicuous, and patients were only allowed to speak when the sister spoke to them. She would stop at the foot of every bed, say a few words to each patient, make a few notes and move on to the next. Even the medical staff stayed away, and remarkably the phone never seemed to ring.

On one particular morning a houseman had removed an indwelling catheter from a patient. As is often the case, the patient felt the need to frequent the toilet. Just before 9.00 a.m. Wendy found the patient crying in her bed, explaining that she badly needed the toilet but was scared to get out of her bed because she would be in trouble with sister.

I told her that was nonsense, and helped her down the ward to the toilet. Of course Sister arrived at the bed and it was empty. She bellowed out. 'Where is this patient?' I walked out to the end of the ward and yelled back that the patient was in the toilet. Sister yelled back at me 'Why?' I yelled back 'What do you usually go to the toilet for?' Sister yelled back at me, 'Get out of my ward now.' I did!

Wendy left and took the rest of the day off. She was very scared and fully expected a visit to the matron's office. This did not happen, possibly because the sister had not informed matron. On duty the next day the sister said nothing – in fact she said nothing to her for the best part of a week. Wendy then had to deliver a message to her, and she proved to be very pleasant. From that point on she was very kind and helpful, although she did not change any of her practices on the ward.

Not all disputes were between the nursing staff. Susan Eardley-Stiff, who trained at the Royal Masonic Hospital, London, was the sister of an antenatal ward in Southampton when a well-known ship's master from one of the major shipping lines arranged for a private room for a woman with an impending delivery. Since he admitted her under his own name it was presumed it was his wife. At the same time his pregnant daughter was admitted and thoughtfully placed in a private room next door. The mother came to visit the daughter and, seeing her surname on the next door, went in to find her husband holding the hand of an obviously pregnant woman she did not know. Susan had to step in to keep them apart.

Other disputes could be caused by the confusion of newborn babies. It was usual to sew name tags on to the babies' wrists. Some mothers were concerned about this, and they would remove them. One Christmas the Lord Mayor came and had his photograph taken with the proud new mothers. But when the mothers returned their babies to the cots two of them thought that they may have taken the wrong ones. This did not result in the trauma it might today, and actually caused some amusement. No definitive test being available the other mothers happily resolved this by confirming that these two mothers had gone to the right cots in the first place.

Dorothy Turner, (née Reynolds) who trained at Boligbroke Hospital, finds the high level of hospital births astonishing – in some districts over 95 per cent.

The problem as I see it is that the more the service encourages women to have births in hospital the more the midwife is deskilled from home delivering. Along with a decline in home births you get an equal decline in midwives who are confident in home deliveries. We seem to have changed into a 'medicalization' of normal births with little or no choice. Caesarean births and other interventions were unusual and only performed in medical emergencies. For decades it has been a midwife-led service, a service that women have always wanted. Fortunately, midwives are now being encouraged to work a balance in the hospital and community so they are more 'rounded' in their experience and should soon be able to offer wider options to mothers. If it is a normal birth there is no reason for involving a doctor therefore no reason for a hospital birth.

She points out the satisfaction of home deliveries, recalling one lady who was pregnant with her ninth child; between nine and thirteen children were not unusual in Beckenham.

I had had a very busy night with about five births and I was tired. Everyone in those days knew where the midwife lived and this little boy knocked at the door, 'Dorothy, come quick, me Mam's in birth.' I thought no, I am too tired, but off I went. I delivered the baby and she was fine. Years later this teenager ran up to me and said, 'My Mam said you delivered me.' I thought, it's time to give in, I must be getting old.

11   Children's Ward Sisters

Order and discipline there must be, or the children will not be happy, but the ward that is tidied up to perfection, in which the little ones look like well drilled soldiers, when liberty is absent, and nothing is out of place, is hardly suggestive of the happy heart of a child.

Catherine Wood, *Nurses' Record*, 1888

It has been an endless battle for doctors and parents to protect infants and children from the ravages of infectious diseases. Up to the twentieth century infant mortality was high and in the poorer families it was intolerable. Scurvy, rickets, smallpox, tuberculosis, and typhus were among the killers, with purging and bleeding the only treatments. A Dr West opened the first hospital for sick children in 1852, at a time when fewer than a third of sick children would be expected to reach adulthood. There were no vaccinations so childhood illnesses such as measles, whooping cough, scarlet fever and rheumatic fever killed, or at the least left sufferers with eye disorders, deafness, heart defects and many other after-effects. There was also tuberculosis. Children did not survive this very well and those who did could be left crippled. One hospital, the Alexandra, catered solely for children with hip conditions caused by TB. Not surprisingly Florence Nightingale thought it an intolerable situation. She felt that a real test for a nurse was whether she could skilfully nurse a sick infant back to health.

In the 1880s a small number of children's hospitals had opened. Lady Superintendent Catherine Wood of the Hospital for Sick Children, London, explained the world of the children's ward. She challenged the regimes for children's wards that were imposed with barely a thought to the needs of the children, making them the cruel dark places often depicted by Dickens. She wrote:

It is the rule to assign a certain defined number of patients to each nurse for whom she is immediately responsible to the sister of the ward. The nurse has the entire care of these patients – she does everything for them, knows all about them . . . The nurse accompanies the sister and the doctor to her charges, and is expected to give an intelligent account of their state and progress.

She believed that sick children did not thrive with a frequent change of attendants, and that the nurse must get to know the child and their ways before she could hope to be successful with them. She added that it was important that in dividing the ward, only as many patients should be assigned to each nurse as she could nurse properly. She also felt that the same regularity and order could not be maintained among the children as on an adult ward. Toys and games were to be as much a part of the treatment as medicine, and the ceaseless chatter and careless distribution of the toys were consistent, she thought, with well-ordered children's wards.

Unfortunately, until early in the twentieth century many children did not enjoy this specialized attention, as they were regularly nursed in adult wards. This practice continued, albeit at much reduced levels, up to recent years. By 1925 there were seven hospitals for sick children approved as training schools in London and fourteen in the provinces. But it was the middle of the 1940s before a registered sick children's nurse qualification was introduced. From then onwards there was a growing awareness of the needs of each child and the parents. It had not been unusual, for example, for a child to be in hospital for six weeks before being allowed visitors. Brenda Beech remembers visitors coming to the sister's office to catch a glimpse of their child through a tiny window, and the children would not see their parents until they were discharged. Sue Clements acknowledges, 'It was thought the children would settle much better. We accepted it then but I now realize that many of the children did not immediately recognize their parents, while the nurses got to know the children so well in that time.' There was therefore always the danger of the nurse acting as surrogate mother to the child in a situation where the child was in hospital for prolonged periods of time. There was also the danger of the nurse wanting to take over from the mother and thinking that she knew what was best for the child.

Sue had begun a four-year combined course in sick children and general nurse training at Great Ormond Street Hospital for Sick Children and the Royal Berkshire Hospitals in 1967. Three of these years were spent with children. With this certificate she had achieved her childhood ambitions of nursing and working with children. She managed to spend most of her nursing years with children, despite a career that included many years in the Queen Alexandra Royal Naval Nursing Service and promotion to deputy matron. Sue found working with children became harder as she got older. She started to recognize the effects of family dynamics on the children she nursed.

Children have always been resilient and I have seen them up the day after major surgery on tricycles. I also recognized more and more how children suffered through attendance at hospitals, and was delighted to be part of the change that recognized the importance of family support. When I started there was restricted visiting and in some cases hardly any visiting. It was wrong but we should not judge with the benefit of hindsight, it was how it was at the time.

Sue identified two special insights a sister needed when working on a children's ward: sensitivity and the anticipation of the child's needs. A nurse could rarely rely on the patient's assistance in letting them know what was wrong. 'A child is generally unable to describe their discomfort,' she explained. 'They may not even be able to describe how uncomfortable they are. Children also live in an immediate world, where responses cannot be delayed. The classic nurses' retort of, "Just a minute" would be meaningless.'

She found that there were lessons to be learned from children, one being that care was needed with the use of language when working with them. She had a young boy on the ward who had been admitted because he had been born without a bladder. He had acute problems with infections, owing to poor urinary control. He constantly followed her about, clinging to her apron, and pressed her to do things for him. She called him, 'my little bully', and he would call her his 'bullyer nurse'. He lived in an orphanage and must have told the nuns about his 'bullyer nurse'. They obviously became somewhat concerned and mentioned their concerns. As she said, 'Seeing the good relationship between the boy and me they were very relieved and very happy. Which is more than can be said for the little boy, who was to be adopted by parents he was obviously not happy with.'

When Mary Hearn was working at an infectious disease hospital in the late 1940s, it was a nurse's duty to go out with the ambulance and the public health officer to bring children into the hospital when they had an infectious disease. A trained fever ambulance nurse had to have the knowledge and courage to open a choking patient's throat quickly, slit the trachea and hold the cut open until they reached the hospital. When she was still a student nurse Mary had to be fully gowned up and wear a mask on such visits before she could enter the child's house. 'What the neighbours thought I do not know! We would be invited into the home, take particulars from the parents and walk off with the child; it was horrendous. Can you imagine how that child felt, and can you imagine that happening today? I hated it.' Gwen Savage, a future senior tutor in paediatric nursing had just such an experience herself. As a child she had suffered from scarlet fever. She remembers the windows of her home being taped over and her room fumigated by a man with a hand pump. To her horror a Black Maria ambulance came to take her away. 'I knew what was happening so I hid in the wardrobe but they still carted me off. The whole thing was worse than a nightmare.' In the ambulance the nurse wrapped her tightly in a blanket and gave whatever comfort she could. When the ambulance arrived at their destination a man in a uniform and peaked cap, the porter, met them and escorted the nurse as she carried Gwen into a big old building, the isolation hospital.

The big problem was always lack of parental contact. 'When there was [contact],' Gwen remembers, 'we had to stand behind a line on the drive with our visitors on another line some distance away, no matter what the weather was like. That continued for about seven weeks.' Other patients told similar stories of parents trying to wave to children through windows, but being moved on as it might upset the child. As one parent said, 'It was as if our child did not belong to us while in there.' Mark Andrews was eleven and his parents could not see him for thirteen weeks apart from over a high wall; he remembers that any parcels for the children had to be thrown over that wall. When the parcels were brought back to the ward, the sister shared out the contents with all the children.

How these experiences affected the children one can only imagine. However, Mary Hearn pointed out: 'To be fair, the thought of introducing further infection into a ward was frightening. The result would have been grim. Prevention was the only option. It was a balance fought between the emotional disturbance of the child and that constant fear of epidemic which informed this approach to care.' The children were nursed in small isolated cubicles but some were more fortunate in being in a four- to six-bed area. There could be as many as twenty to thirty beds in a ward. Fresh air was the treatment of choice for any chest complaint and so these children would find themselves joining others on the 'sun parlour'. This was a bit of a euphemism, especially in the north: it would mean being pushed out on to a very cold and windy veranda. On many occasions Mary found the working conditions distressing.

In the winter we would be in the room sorting the child out and then have to go outside to go to the next child, so we were in and out of the cold all day. We nurses often suffered from chapped hands, it being the days before disposable nappies. At the end of a walkway there was a big coffer and into this would be dumped all the nappies. The sister was in the central area and rarely ventured into the outside. Although we all loved working with the children and our hearts went out to them, none of us really enjoyed the conditions of work.

Alice Ashworth described a typical morning on the children's ward when working at the Northern General Hospital, Sheffield, in 1940. The night staff gave out the breakfast, recorded the temperatures and pulse and gave the children their baths. The day staff came on at

8.00 a.m. Alice described the sister as a wonderful lady who would always go round the ward to see the children and check on them. She said, 'To a waking child we nurses must have seemed strange with our tall white caps tied under our chins, starched aprons and dresses down to our ankles. Sister had a fancy white cap with well-starched wings and wore a blue uniform.' Everyone moved briskly around the ward, straightening beds, tucking in bedding, stoking the coal fires, especially when the big business was the morning round by the matron, a formidable woman in blue.

Matron would normally 'sweep' into a ward attended by an administration sister who took on a very efficient and firm manner. But on the children's ward she ensured that she spoke to each child and was aware of the different approach she needed. We nurses were busy throughout this time on menial tasks, happy to be busy during this normally formidable visitation from above. The children were blissfully unaware of the importance of the visit.

Working on night duty Alice found the work very demanding.

I was working on a whooping cough ward, and believe me it was hard work. Among all my other duties I had to count how many times a child coughed in the night. I had no help and I did not have a break. Night Sister would come round twice a night and check all the patients and see that I was keeping a proper record.

For almost all children preparation for operating day was a very frightening experience and, in the days before premedication, entry into the annexe of the operating theatre could be highly intimidating. The staff in their gowns and gloves were bad enough, but then they were introduced to the ether mask. It came over the nose and mouth and the sweet and sickly smell of gas would always be remembered. At least by the time they were taken into theatre they were spared the sight of trays of gleaming instruments, hissing sterilizers, clanging metal trolleys, gas cylinders and the dreadful smell of iodine. On return to the ward the child would invariably be sick, which was particularly discomforting if a chest or stomach operation had been performed.

Following their operation there would be the dreaded treatment area. It consisted of a treatment table, a sterilizer and porcelain sink. Following the doctor's round, child after child would be led very reluctantly to this area. Helen Baig sadly remembers being one of three nurses who held a child while the fourth nurse did the dressing.

It is something I never could get used to. I remember all the poor children, I am sure they could never quite understand why one minute we were so kind to them and then we would put them through the most awful pain. After a mastoidectomy the patient was given a light anaesthetic for the first dressing. I do remember those at the private hospital got a mild anaesthetic for the first two or three dressing changes.

The dressing of the wounds entailed the removal of the ribbon gauze from the cavity. This was soaked with saline before they could ease it out; it was never painless. After being cleaned with peroxide the wound was repacked with iodoform ribbon gauze. The most frequent cases would have sticks of silver nitrate inserted into the wound, which caused excessive discomfort and the child would scream throughout the treatment. One trick a sister used was to have a child relaxed by the fire and then she would ask if she could look at the scar, initially easing the dressing back. Then she would rip it off, believing that a moment's pain was better than what she believed was the slower, more painful agony of removing it a little at a time.

In the late 1950s there was a growing recognition of the importance of children being nursed by those with a registered sick children nurse qualification. Previously a ward sister was often the only person on a ward with this qualification. She had to guide the new student nurses and junior doctors, as many of them had had no experience of looking after young children. Children's wards were usually mixtures of infectious diseases, general surgery, genito-urinary surgery (reconstruction of deformities of the genitalia) and medical conditions such as meningitis and bronchitis. Unique to children's nursing was the fact that a child could be on the ward from a few days old, through their childhood and into adulthood. The nurse would get very close to them and their parents.

Jean Bajnath (née Hussain) pointed out that up to the 1980s the doctor's word on the children's wards possibly carried too much weight. Nursing children had its unique problems and she feels this was not always considered.

Young children deteriorate much quicker than adults do; time is of the essence. The majority of new doctors have not had experience of working with children. For example, if a child needs an intravenous infusion and an inexperienced doctor cannot find a vein after two or three attempts, then the nurse has to step in as the vein will collapse. The doctor would not like it, but as nurses we had a duty to the child. It was not a criticism of the doctor; it was to protect the child.

It was the same with the increasing use of drugs.

For children, a nurse has to be extremely watchful of any dosage prescribed. In adult nursing milligrams are mostly used, whereas with children micrograms are more readily prescribed. When administering these drugs it is a nurse's responsibility to check the dosage. If the nurse follows a prescription and the dosage is wrong the nurse is accountable.

Norma Clacey remembers being perpetually scared of the sister of the children's ward. She was devoted to the physical care of the children, but she did not always understand their emotional needs, or the emotional needs of her nurses. She most certainly did not consider that anyone else could possibly look after the children as well as she could, and she was not keen for young student nurses to be responsible for a child. On the basis of this experience Norma vowed that she would be as aware as she could be of emotional needs, particularly when the time came for her to be sister of a children's ward herself. She was once blanket-bathing a young girl who was very depressed. The girl owned a horse that she was very fond of, which was being cared for by her friend. It was all she could think about. Norma suggested that the friend bring the horse in its horse-box to the hospital car park. The girl instantly perked up and was delighted by the idea. The day arrived and so did the horse. An amused switchboard member informed her that the horse was on its way. Wheeling the young lady down the corridor to the entrance she could hardly believe her eyes. The girl's friend was halfway up the corridor leading the horse. 'Well, the scene of this horse slipping and sliding all over the polished corridor floor was wonderful, I expected it any minute to collapse with all its legs spread apart. But it was worth the effort, the girl was thrilled and delighted; not sure that the corridor maid was quite so delighted.'

We nurses were not constrained by health and safety regulations and there was not the consideration to cross infection then. We felt we were sufficiently aware of cleanliness issues to manage such problems, so a popular gift to children's wards were large, fluffy, cuddly animals, and with these my nurses would provide backrests for the children. The children would get tremendous comfort from snuggling into them.

Also on the ward was a doll's house and she was fascinated watching the children rearrange the furniture.

A few of these children had only lived in flats and they would arrange the furniture on one floor. Some had never seen a man and woman in bed together and this would be reflected by the use of dolls. This was more noticeable when working with children following the break-up of marriage. Young children would come into hospital following an accident and quite often have the parents squabbling.

She found she had few difficulties with the children. They would come in, have a bath, have their hair washed and be quickly settled. '[But] one particular child came in and we bathed and scrubbed him and his parents came to visit; walking up and down the ward they failed to recognize him. When he came in to us his hair was a mousy brown and when we washed it, it had turned blond, it was extraordinary.'

The most distressing occasion in all nursing is death, and the death of a child is utterly heartbreaking. It is particularly hard for junior nurses, who are often young themselves, not to get emotionally involved. For many the only experience of death may have been the loss of a pet, and it is hard for them to come to terms with such an untimely loss as a child. So a death was a problem the sister had to be aware of. Many rightly or wrongly dealt with it by keeping nurses busy, tidying cupboards, cleaning the sluice room or other such chores, ostensibly to keep the nurses' minds off the trauma. If any counselling was given, the sister gave it; in-house counselling was something for the future.

When Joan Page was training at the Queen's Hospital for Children in the 1940s, laying-out following the death of a child was always done with due reverence and care. They had shrouds of a stiff cotton material with tapes to draw up and tie at the neck and wrists, giving a frilled effect rather reminiscent of choirboy's surplice.

> We took pride in making the child and the cubicle look as perfect at possible. We would fold the hands together and place at least one white flower in them. Often of course we would not have any on the ward and would run round to all the other wards until we had managed to obtain one; they were always willing to help.

Thus it was that most parents saw their child looking as peaceful as possible with all signs of treatment removed from the room.

'When the child was taken to the mortuary,' Joan said, 'we would carry it in our arms wrapped in a blanket so if any other children saw us they wouldn't realize what had happened.' One nurse was carrying such a child along the corridor to the mortuary when a visitor asked if she could look at the baby. 'My heart nearly stopped,' she said. 'But not wanting to get into an explanation about the child's death I uncovered enough of the face to satisfy the lady, then carried on to the mortuary.'

Later, when she was a sister on the children's ward at the Royal Free Hospital, Joan had one child, Tommy, who had been admitted many times with osteomyelitis. Tommy was six years old and like many of the children admitted he was from a very poor area. The boys used to stand on the balcony and collect bus registration numbers. Joan recalls, 'Tommy was not as quick as the others, so I would help him when I could, writing down numbers for all I was worth.' Tommy went home but clearly missed the contact with the other children and the security of the ward and the nurses. It was likely that he was left to fend for himself on the streets.

His little face would peer round the ward door asking if he could come in. He would play with the toys and the children, have plenty of ice cream and jelly and I would then take him by the hand down to the lift to the front of the hospital and make him promise to ask a policeman to cross him over the busy King's Cross Road.

Mary Hearn remembers working on a children's ward where the standards were impeccable, but 'the sister was a dragon of a woman – faultless with the children, awful to us.' When she was on night duty, Mary and her colleagues had to look after six babies in cubicles and twenty toddlers. Each ward had a first-, second-, and third-year student between them. The senior nurse had the six babies to look after, acute cases of pyloric-stenosis (stricture of the pyloric orifice) and other abdominal conditions. It was her job to feed and care for them. Mary and one other student nurse had the twenty toddlers to look after. The sister would come on duty at 8.00 a.m. and the ward would have to be perfect. All the children and their cots would have to be spick and span and the children had to have their hair done. 'The girls had bows in their hair,' she said. 'Can you imagine the work this entailed? If any child was found wet, there was the devil to pay. We would have gone round sitting them all on potties prior to her coming on duty, praying, please go!' On arrival sister would go into the toddler area and take off all the babies' nappies and check for red bottoms.

Of course the children were all crying for their mothers first thing in the morning, but undeterred she would do this ritualistic examination, it was pandemonium as you can imagine. She only had to find one problem and it meant staying on to sort it out, then we would be in trouble with the night sister, who was waiting to check us into the dining room.

On night duty during the Second World War Grace Bartlett had twenty babies to look after and each was issued with a gas mask.

It was a sort of canvas thing that you pushed the baby into head first until their little faces appeared in the perspex bit at the top; their arms and legs you had to push in the bag then draw up and fasten it. There was one under each cot. Thank goodness I did not have to use it; how could any one person have ever managed to get twenty babies into these things if there had been an attack?

Managing with a ward full of babies could be challenging at night without such added problems. Alice Carr remembers:

On the children's ward we could have a ward full of gastro-enteritis so it was a never-ending round of nappies and feeds. The bottles of feed would be placed in warm water in big crates. I would go round to each cot and prop the bottle with a napkin so the baby could feed, and then I had to wind them. That was all you could do, it was exhausting.

A difficult problem nurses could face on children's wards was the receiving of presents. It was often hard to say no, but that is a rule in nursing that has not changed. Judith Clark was working on a children's ward when a little girl of nine was admitted. She had been dancing with her sister, twirling around, when her skirt caught light from an open fire, burning her very badly. It was a distressing experience for Judith, who had to dress the burns, in the 1940s these took a great deal of time. With the unique nurse-child relationship on a children's ward she also had a great deal of contact with the parents. Sadly the girl died. Some time later the parents came to her on the ward with an expensive gift to thank her for all she had done. She should have refused, 'but how could I say no? I thought they had been hurt enough. I told the ward sister and she reported it to the hospital secretary. I had to go to his office with Matron, but they said they would accept it this time but not to do it again, and returned the gift to me.'

The care of children has developed enormously and made major advances with the diagnosis of illnesses, their treatments and the emotional care of child and family. Since the 1980s paediatric palliative care has developed alongside – though separate from – the hospice movement, the first paediatric hospice being Helen House in Oxford, which opened in 1982. Beginning in paediatric oncology, specialist nurses have developed their skills and are now providing advice on symptom management and support to the family.

12   Casualty and Out-patient Sisters

It is always more difficult to teach others to do anything than to
do it one's self – it requires great patience, pressed as they
[sisters] are, to get the actual work done.

Miss Crossland, letter to Florence Nightingale, 1876

Casualty and out-patient departments were historically combined
under one sister, except at very large hospitals. The receiving rooms
where patients waited for treatment at the turn of the nineteenth
century were usually large halls teeming with people; there was no
appointment system. They had to be patient, and in those days they
mostly were. They were treated free but the price was tolerance.
Waiting times could be very long, sometimes many hours.

The extraordinary techniques of bandaging were learned in the
nursing school and the accident department. Bandages were made of
unbleached calico, flannel, or domett. The most widely used was the
roller bandage, about 6–8 yards in length and from 1–6 inches wide.
Bandaging was quite an art, and nurses would take great pride in
their skill. The rules were to fix the bandage by two or three turns
over the limb, to bandage from below upwards and from within
outwards over the front of the limb, to use firm but equable pressure
throughout, to let each succeeding turn overlap the preceding one by
two-thirds, to let the crossings and reverses be in one neat line
towards the front of the limb, and to complete by fixing the bandage
securely with a safety pin. There were also spiral bandages, reverse
spirals, figure-of-eights, spicas, capelines for the head, the many-
tailed and the T-bandage for retaining dressings on the perineum (the
area between the thighs). Other associated equipment would be slings
for arms, pads for splints and sandbags to support fractured limbs.

Antiseptic solutions of various strengths were always available, as were eucalyptus, vaseline or boracic ointment, iodoform, prepared cat-gut ligatures, silk ligatures, drainage tubes, oiled silk protective, antiseptic gauze, thin mackintosh cloth, loose antiseptic gauze, gauze bandages and safety-pins. A spray producer would also be in readiness. This steam apparatus consisted of a large glass bottle containing a solution of carbolic acid. Water, kept on the boil, enabled a mixture of steam and carbolic to be produced as a fine spray of antiseptic. Cupping was the main treatment at the turn of the nineteenth century and when the hospital cupper retired (which was rare) or died there would be urgent requests from the medical staff to train another.

Towards the end of the nineteenth century, casualty departments had a sister with the title of Sister of Massage and Electricity. Most major hospitals would employ at least one. At the end of the nineteenth century massage and low-frequency electricity were very popular therapies. Many nurses went to Europe, in particular Germany and Sweden, in order to learn the techniques. Courses were expensive, costing around 50 guineas. In Britain, the best schools to learn massage techniques were thought to be the National Hospital, London, and the Nurses' Club in the Strand. At these institutions the cost of training could be somewhere in the region of 5–15 guineas.

Massage was used extensively in casualty departments and also for long-term patients. At its height it was thought to be beneficial for acute patients in relaxing the stiffness and 'fixation' of joints after injury and in chronic conditions for the relief of constipation, particularly in bedridden patients. However, the extensive use of massage fell out of fashion after the First World War as too expensive considering the limited number of patients a nurse could work on in a day. Electricity was used to stimulate damaged muscles and nerves from either acute trauma or prolonged inactivity from continuous bed care. Coming direct from a multi-cell battery, either continuous (galvanic) or interrupted (faradic) current was used. It was thought that cases of paralysis from spinal nerve disease were some of the main beneficiaries. Later the physiotherapist would assume responsibility for many of these activities.

At the beginning of the twentieth century, the sister and nurses took on higher levels of responsibility in casualty departments than anywhere else. Rarely had nurses given injections, as this was still the domain of medical staff, but in the casualty department boundaries blurred and nurses were often called upon to give hypodermic injections as well as suture simple wounds. The First World War accelerated cross-domain work. Nurses proved that they could take on far more responsibility than they had previously been allowed. Following the First World War nurses routinely gave most of the injections.

A particular problem during the Second World War was the extended blackout. An absence of street lighting and hooded car headlamps made accidents more numerous and more severe. This blackout also produced unique problems for medical staff and nurses. Until the hospitals acquired all the blackout curtains they needed, nursing staff had to work with low wattage blue lighting. This was a problem on any ward, but particularly in the casualty department. Here there was an increase in the level and severity of accidents to deal with. Major bleeds illuminated with dim blue light were particularly difficult to manage.

Following the war nurses began to do most of the suturing at many provincial casualty departments, as medical staff did not have the time. Unfortunately this could involve too much responsibility for junior nurses. David Turner was a student nurse working in a small casualty department in the early 1950s when a young boy was admitted. He had fallen from a bicycle and badly lacerated his face. One wound, a deep gash, stretched from the corner of his mouth up into his cheek. The doctor and sister were both very busy, and David was directed to suture the boy's face.

To be honest I did not use enough local anaesthetic to completely deaden his wound and so when I started suturing it must have hurt like hell. I carried on as if I knew what I was doing, but I know I did not use as many sutures as I should have done, to save him from any more suffering. I did not see him when the sutures were taken out and I still wonder what sort of scar I left him with. I knew it was wrong and I should have refused, but in those days you tended to follow what you had been directed to do. It would now be a very skilled cosmetic job.

Tom Noakes remembers how many men would come into casualty at the Royal Hospital, Wolverhampton, in the 1950s with distended bladders. Too embarrassed to talk about their 'problem' it had to be a crisis for them to seek help. They were diagnosed with renal retention and the nurse would catheterize them. The nurses would also pass gastric tubes and put in intravenous cannulas to set up drips. They also did all the plastering of fractures in the department; sometimes an orderly would assist. Plaster of Paris and Gipsona were used. It was also the nurse on night duty in casualty at many hospitals, and certainly the Royal Hospital, who would certify death and carry out last offices for the patient.

Tom remembers one patient coming in with terrible pain in his ear. The doctor examined him and found no problem, but the patient continued to complain to Tom that he was in dreadful pain. 'I decided to look in the ear myself and could actually see something move. I got a pair of crocodile forceps and low and behold, I pulled out a moth, alive.' He also wishes he had a pound for every industrial staple he has removed. Near the hospital was a box factory that used 2 inch long staples with 1 inch teeth. These became embedded in arms and legs and were very painful to remove.

On night duty Tom was in sole charge, with doctors being called in only on his advice. One night, just after the book *Doctor in the House* was published, it was initially quiet, and Tom was reading it.

I had just got started when all hell was let loose, police, ambulances and patients seemed to arrive at once. Collins fairground staff were in a coach, and a lorry had crashed into them. The driver was drunk or, as we would say then, mentally confused. There were at least ten passengers with fractured skulls, many had multiple internal and limb injuries. I was on my own until a doctor arrived and then Miss Grey, the matron. She said, 'What do you want me to do child?' She called everyone child because she could not remember names. I pointed out a patient who had to go to X-ray and off she went with him. By now I was joined by two of the night sisters. We were stopping bleeding, ensuring clear airways, and infusing with saline. While all this was happening theatre was being prepared.

Barbara Hare remembers treatments being very primitive compared with today. 'Varicose ulcers did not heal for months, if ever. The only treatment in the early fifties was Viscopaste on a wet bandage which hardened into a thin plaster-of-Paris-type dressing.' Each week this was cut off and another bandage applied. Beryl Varilone was one of many nurses who cut off such a bandage to find dozens of maggots squirming on the floor. 'This sounds repulsive, but when I looked at the leg the flesh was completely red and clean. I do not know how the fly got in, but I do know it was a horrible job cleaning up the floor.' This was not particularly unusual but always unpleasant for the nurse and patient.

Trephining was one of the most immediately rewarding but at the same time hazardous tasks in casualty. Many injuries to fingers entailed blood collecting under the nail. Relieving it was a simple though unsavoury procedure. Alice Forbes pointed out the dangers.

When I was shown the technique it entailed heating the end of a metal paper clip on a burner and when it was red hot using this to pierce the nail. Good advice was to hold the finger well away as blood would fly when the nail was pierced. But it was a satisfying procedure as it afforded immediate relief to the patient; it also caused fainting. So after explaining to the patient what was to be done it was best carried out with the patient sat down; the biggest men fell the heaviest.

For sisters in casualty and out-patients departments the move from direct in-patient care to a less hands-on post could have its own problems. Rita Hobbs was the sister of out-patients and casualty at King's College Hospital, Norwood, in the late 1940s. The departments were very busy; as well as dealing with emergencies they also handled the removal of tonsils, syringing of ears, routine changes of dressing, the removal of sutures and cleaning ulcerated wounds. As sister, she enjoyed the challenge of organizing and running the department but felt a little removed from direct nursing care. Until she settled she spent a great deal of her off-duty time helping on the in-patient wards to keep her hand in.

When I started nursing they really were accident wards; intensive care units were many years away. We did not have the sophisticated equipment of today so our immediate principle was to limit further damage. As I recall, my junior nurses were far more involved than when I started. We had been little more than handmaidens to the various specialities and senior nurses, we were virtually there to set the tables with the instruments laid out, and the roof would fall in if you got any of it wrong.

In this post Rita could for the first time be non-resident. 'For the first time in my life I could close the place at night, go home to my own room and not worry; it seemed like a new luxury.' Casualty had reduced staffing at night and when there was an emergency it was agreed that she would be called out to return to the hospital and take responsibility herself. She came to enjoy the constant turnover of patients. She was aware that to a new nurse every day was different in casualty, a constant challenge, but to an experienced nurse the most acute emergencies had a sense of routine about them. 'Most of them were a repetition of previous emergencies,' she said. 'With these we would require immediate admission but unlike today with bed managers we would liaise with the accident, medical or surgical wards and get the patients transferred.'

Marion Dyson spent twenty-four years in charge of the out-patient department at Huddersfield Royal Infirmary. Here she worked on all the departments, particularly chaperoning examinations by consultants and following up treatments. Nurses took blood, as well as swabs for microscopic investigation. They also did the diagnostic work on the microscope. 'It was such satisfying and rewarding work for nurses,' she said. 'The patients were not handed from department to department, and the nurses were directly involved in all the stages of investigation, diagnosis and treatment.'

Patients' behaviour in those days was less confrontational than it sometimes is today. Janice Bell says:

> We had observation beds at the Liverpool Royal Infirmary so we had the option of keeping patients overnight. We did not of course have the drug problem in the 1950s – drunks, yes, but rarely did we have to call the police. I guess even when drunk they were more respectful of us. We did have very good relations with the police; they used to visit the department regularly. There was a little office where they would have a cup of

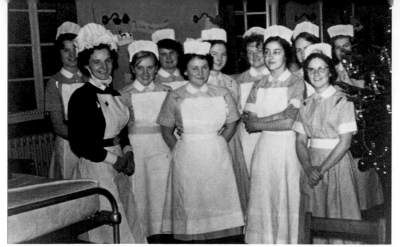

Sister Daphne Bunney (later Fallows)
with the staff of Victoria ward,
Hydestile, Godalming, 1959

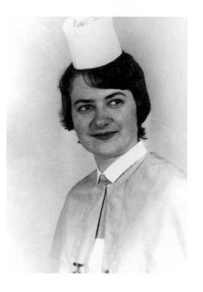

Liz Carter knew all the 'pranks' the
nurses got up to when she was
night sister at the Royal Masonic
Hospital, Hammersmith, 1973

Charge Nurse Roy Stallard (*back row, far right*) at the prizegiving at
Wolverhampton Eye Infirmary, 1959, where Matron Jones (*centre*)
actively encouraged male nurses

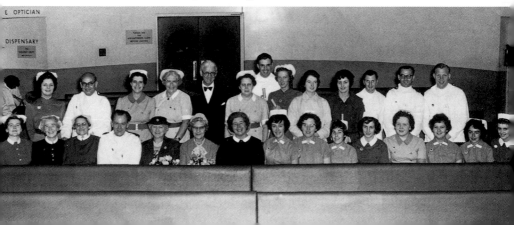

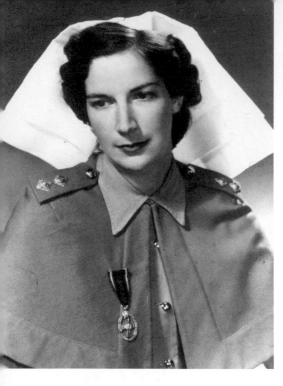

Joan Pease, nursing sister in the uniform of Queen Alexandra's Royal Army Nursing Corps, 1946

Sister Marion Dyson in the 1960s preparing the trolley for the important role of serving lunch to patients at Huddersfield Royal Infirmary

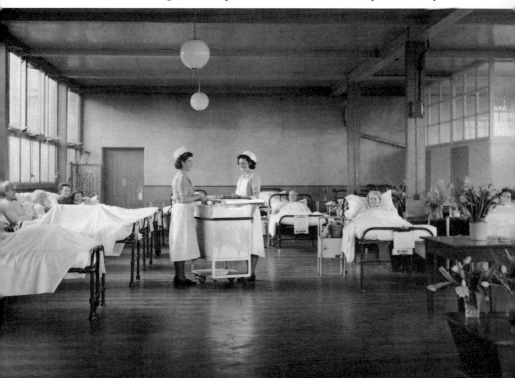

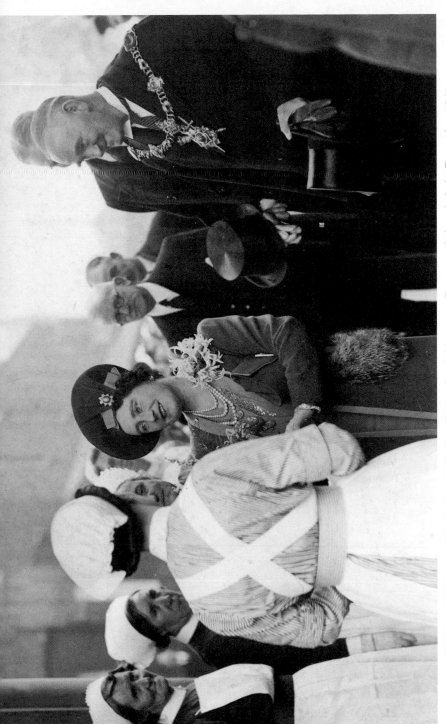

Visit by HM Queen Elizabeth and Sir Dan Daley, Lord Mayor, to Portsmouth hospitals in December 1941

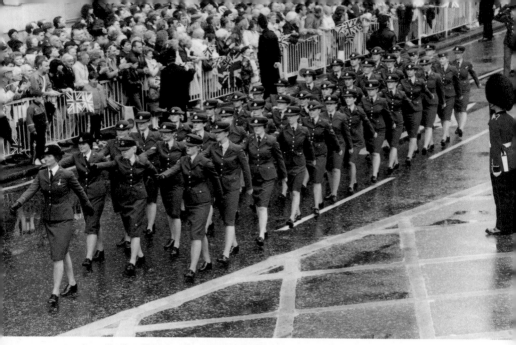

Angela Scofield leading the parade of Princess Mary's Royal Air Force
Sisters at the Gulf War Commemoration, 1991

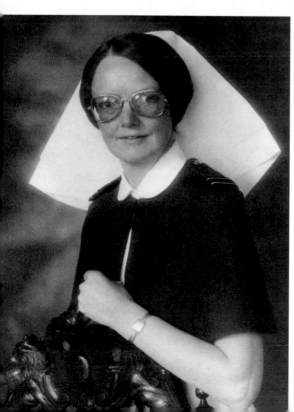

Angela Scofield, one of the
first sisters in the uniform of
flight lieutenant in Princess
Mary's Royal Air Force, 1980

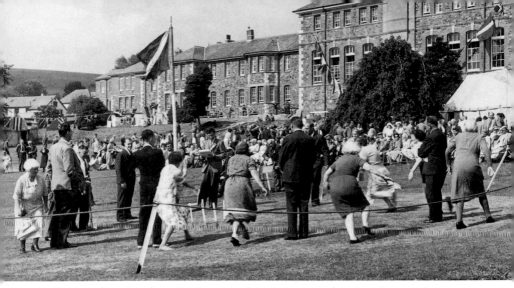

Both staff and patients having great fun at the annual patients' sports day
at Moorhaven Mental Hospital, Plymouth, 1952

Aileen Gardner (*right*) enjoys taking care of the new Christmas babies in
the premature baby unit, 1956. Sister would allow her nurses to wear
tinsel in their hats but she wouldn't wear it herself

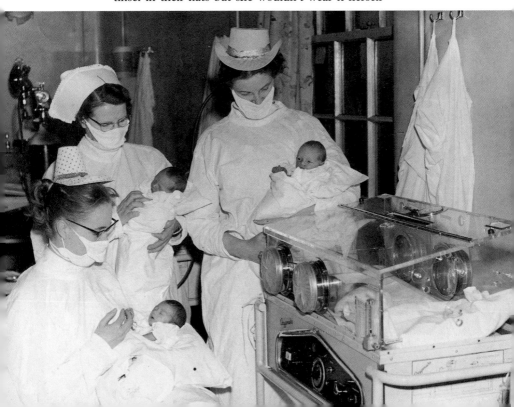

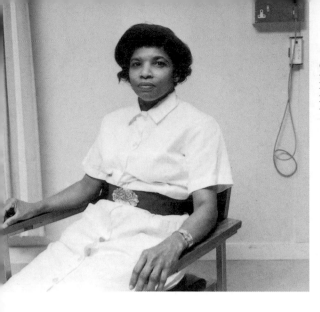

Clinical teacher Lynette Patterson at Queen Mary's Hospital for children, London, 1972

Sister Kay Riley leading daily prayers on Elizabeth Ward, St Thomas's Hospital, 1960. She continued this daily activity until her retirement in 1987

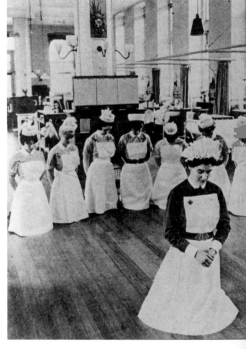

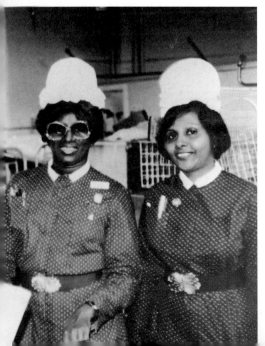

Sisters Janet Campbell and Seta Singh on the elderly care ward and in the uniform of South Western Hospital, London, 1979

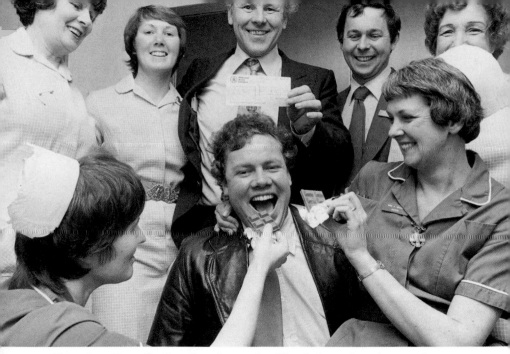

Sister Ann Grose feeding chocolate to Ian Hough (porter) at the casualty department, Queen Alexandra Hospital, Cosham, following a weight-loss fund-raising event. Sister Denise Rock (*front left*) assists, 1981

(*Left to right*) Midwife Jennie Vinall, Matron Margaret Pettigrew, Avril Williamson (later Vincent) and, seated, Mrs Pettigrew (matron's mother) at Blake House, Gosport, 1966

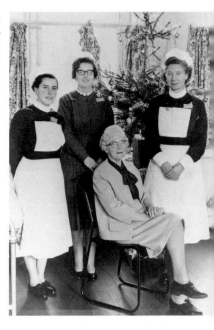

Dorothy Turner (*far right*) and Cynthia Braithwaite (*second from left*) in nurse training at Bolingbroke Hospital, 1963

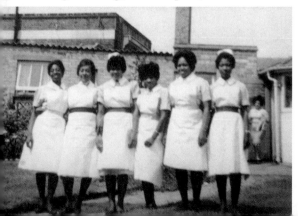

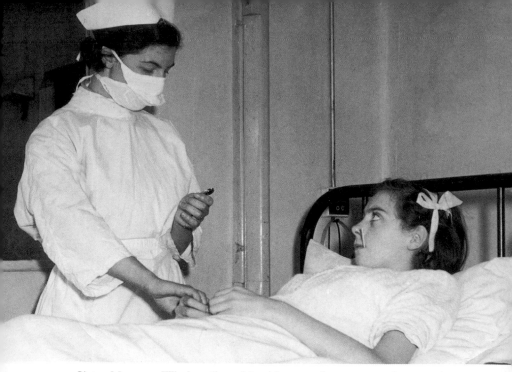

Sister Margaret Window (later Morris) gowned up to attend to a patient with TB meningitis at Rush Green Hospital, c. 1957

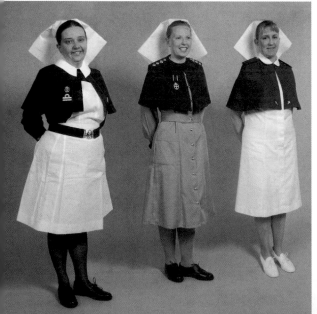

Tri-service nursing sisters, Lieutenant Maria Rea (Navy), Captain Lyndsey Hunter (Army), and Flight Lieutenant Helene Martin (Air Force) in traditional uniform, 2004. These uniforms will be retained for ceremonial use only, when they are replaced by modern nursing dress tea, and just their presence was enough to settle any problems we might have.

Joan Jenkins was working as a sister in the casualty department at St George's Hospital, London, in 1939 when the matron approached her and said, 'I have always provided a sister to attend the hop-pickers' camp in Kent to deal with any accidents and emergencies; would you consider this for a month?' She would be in charge of both the casualty and dispensary tents. 'Not only was I told to be in my St George's uniform at all times in the camp,' Joan said, 'I was also told I had to travel in full uniform.' When she arrived, there must have been a hundred huts in one large area near the village of Yalding, Kent, where the hop-pickers lived for the time of the harvesting.

The gypsies were also there, the real gypsies, not the travellers of today. I nursed many of their children who had pneumonia. I had a surgery every morning where I had to do all the incisions and suturing – the local GP certainly did not expect to do this – and I diagnosed scarlet fever by candlelight; it was a wonderful experience.

There were some Voluntary Aid Detachment (VADs) women who were nearly all debutantes, wanting to do their bit for the war effort. All the doors to the huts were open, day and night.

We nurses lived in the village hall and never thought to lock a door. The people in Yalding were incredibly hospitable. They would invite me and the VADs to their houses, leave their doors unlocked, with a glass of sherry, a piece of cake and a bath ready for us. Then we would come away and just shut the door.

The following year Joan was again asked to work with the VADs, this time at the territorial camp at Burley in the New Forest.

My friend and I, who was also a sister, ran the casualty and camp hospital. It was a tented camp. General Buller's granddaughter, Millicent Buller, was the head of the VAD section. When we returned to London she invited my friend and me to lunch at her Knightsbridge flat. We both wore hats for the occasion but were surprised when Miss Buller came out of her room in her own house with a hat on – because it was correct to lunch with a hat on.

On the night of VE Day, Billie Cullen (née Bisland) joined the line of nurses outside the night sister's office at Radcliffe Hospital to be allocated her work for the night – this event was known at the hospital as the slave market. She was sent to help out in the casualty department. Heralding the end of the war in Europe, Oxford, like most of the major cities, was receiving both military and civilian casualties. This victory celebration was like no other. Pent up feelings were at last released and with it many revellers suffered severe accidents. People fell from lamp posts, telegraph poles and other vantage points to which they had climbed to watch others parading and dancing in the streets. Some also fell through shop windows, causing dreadful lacerations. The repair of fractures and the suturing of wounds were the main concerns of the medical and nursing staff. Later in the night alcohol poisoning was not unusual, so stomach pumps were very much in evidence.

Margaret Webster worked in Casualty at the Royal Hospital in Sheffield in the 1950s.

Here we had plenty of drunks but these were easily dealt with and it was very rare to call for assistance; they respected us as nurses. I do not recall there being high numbers of road traffic accidents or cardiac arrests in those days, more congestive cardiac, probably because of the smoke from the steel works, and renal failures.

There were many injuries from rock climbing, courtesy of Derbyshire's geology, mainly multiple fractures and severe skin lacerations. There were also many injuries from the steel works: burns from molten metal that would literally go through the bone, crush injuries and amputations. Small splinters of steel caused eye injuries and as long as the splinter had not penetrated too deeply the nurses could remove them. The eye would be dyed with Flourecine, a bluish-yellow colour, to show the splinter, and it would be removed with a pair of tweezers. One morning a week at this casualty department was designated 'tramps' morning. Margaret explained, 'These poor mendicants would come in to have their feet washed and their toenails clipped. For some reason many would have septic fingers so these were also treated and their overall health checked. They were very grateful for the attention.' They were also grateful for the plate of food and drink that the nurses scrounged from the wards for them.

When Brenda Beech was working at the Eye Infirmary, Wolverhampton, a patient presented himself in the accident department. The charge nurse took some personal details before asking what the problem was. The patient replied, 'It's not me, it's my budgie.' With this he took a small box from his overcoat pocket, opened it and there was the budgie. He explained that its eyesight was so poor it kept missing its perch in the cage. The charge nurse duly put a couple of drops in its eyes and the man left much happier.

The first days working in casualty can be extremely traumatic. For Ian Hough they were the worst of his life. After a time in the entertainment business, he switched to hospital work and was on a three-week contract at Queen Alexandra Hospital, Cosham, as a porter. Starting at 8.30 a.m. he was instructed to go to the casualty department. He arrived just as there was a crisis. He was very confused with all that was going on and when there was a shout of, 'Porter, Porter', he thought, 'That must be me!' Then the staff started to ask him to get various things of which he had no idea.

I just went with the flow. Then an ambulance pulled in to the reception area and the doors flew open. One of the crew said, 'Take this'; it was a plastic bag. Not having any idea what to do, I looked in the bag, which I feel now I probably should not have done, and there was a woman's leg. I had never seen or been involved with anything so horrific in my life. I had to sit outside to recover my composure.

Realizing what had happened, Sister Ann Grose (née Chick) gave support to her new staff member and took him for a cup of tea to calm his nerves. At lunchtime the nursing officer, also aware of what had happened, took him to the local pub, which he found full of doctors and nurses, including some of the staff he had worked with that morning. Three weeks later, and a stone and a half lighter, he was asked if he would like the post full time. Nervously he went to the interview. There were only the nursing officer and sister there, and he got the job. Twenty-six years later, reflecting his theatrical days and his sense of humour, he now sports a badge with the title of 'Consultant Trolleyologist'.

One event he has never got used to, however, is sudden death, particularly the death of toddlers and babies.

Some of the accidents we see are dreadful, but because of the support of the team I first worked with I learned to cope. What I like is that although I am 'only' a porter my opinion is respected as much as anyone else's. When the doctor thinks there is no hope for a patient he checks with the whole team and that includes me.

Ann Grose had always wanted to nurse. As a child, her dolls were noted for the flaking paint on their faces, caused by 'so much medicine', and their arms and legs were forever being bandaged; they were never allowed to get better before the next accident. Her main interest was in casualty work, and she achieved her ambition after passing her final state registration examinations in 1961 at Taunton and Somerset Hospital. After a break to have her family, she was appointed Sister Casualty back at this hospital. As it was on the main route to the West Country, she would see holidaymakers eager to get to their destinations, who had driven long distances without a break and been involved in dreadful accidents. Casualty received the injured and on occasions whole families would be brought in.

Apart from these sadly routine accidents she recalls another traumatic experience.

On one occasion we had a gentleman admitted whose mentally retarded son had stabbed him with a large, curved bagging or sacking needle. X-rays showed that the needle was embedded in the heart so a medical decision was made to move him immediately to Bristol, some fifty miles away.

Being sister of the unit, Ann went with the patient in the ambulance.

Her only instruction was to try to stop the needle moving. Much to her consternation, it did start to move, despite the padding around it. The ambulance pulled to the side of the road and the doctor at Taunton was radioed. He could only advise them to get to Bristol as fast as possible and make sure the needle stayed where it was. Arriving at Frenchay Hospital, Bristol, it was with great relief that Ann handed the patient over to the waiting medical crew. The needle was removed under safer conditions in the operating theatre, and the patient thankfully survived.

Later Ann moved to a city hospital casualty department. There it was noticeable that the types of incidents were very different. One example was overdosing; whereas an overdose in the rural area was likely to be due to an accidental intake of agricultural fluids, in the city it was far more likely to be a deliberate act of self harm.

Audrey Chambers believes that:

The world was very different before the 1960s. I think people were more courteous and considerate to nurses. Up to the late 1970s for a sister of a casualty department it had been very much hands on. The patients seemed to have a better under-standing of the purpose of casualty and their demands on us were thought to be more reasonable. For the most part they seemed to know what was appropriate with minor injuries treated at home or at the local family doctor. By the late 1980s we were seeing more patients and the demands were greater.

To deal with these changes, casualty departments were renamed acci-dent and emergency. It was hoped that this would educate the public into recognizing the new emphasis of accidents and emergencies only; it did not work. Attitudes were changing and demands for more immediate attention for the most minor complaints continued to grow.

Jean Bajnath was the occupational health nurse in the dockyard at Portsmouth in the 1970s. Her twelve years there were as near to casu-alty nursing as one could get, but without the equipment and back-up.

I never did know what the day would hold. Heart attacks,

165

strokes, diabetic comas and even suicide. There were many falls, machine injuries, eye injuries or blast injuries. You had to go and attend these injuries and apart from the first aider you were the one expected to deal with the situation. The dockyard had twenty thousand workers, so whenever a situation arose you were always closely observed. It was very frightening and stressful, I do not think that in the twelve years there I ever really got used to that. You learnt on the job so to speak, there were no courses on what to do.

She was hardly ever given a full account of the accident prior to attending.

I was called to one where a fork-lift truck had turned over and crushed someone beneath. When I got there acid from the damaged battery was dripping on to the injured person. I did not know what to do. I could not get under the vehicle, as there was the danger it might slip again, but I had to protect him from further injury. The truck needed lifting but it was late so there were no crane drivers available so I had to call the fire brigade. In the meantime I got a canvas sheet and managed to get that over him to protect him from the acid.

Roy Stallard was the charge nurse of Maclaren Accident and Emergency Ward at the Royal Hospital, Wolverhampton. On the ward were thirty emergency beds for men, which would often be increased to forty. On Friday and Saturday nights men would be admitted from casualty with perforated ulcers. Men would also have to admit they really did have a bladder problem, when it became enlarged and they could not pass urine. Their bladders required slow emptying to avoid shock. They were affectionately known as the 'bladder daddies' (enlarged prostates). Many who were admitted to this ward would be young men with fractures from sport or motor-bike injuries. They became bored with little to do. Transferred to an orthopaedic ward they had many weeks in hospital, as bone repair in traction meant a long stay in bed and slow recovery. It was also heavy nursing requiring a great deal of lifting and tugging. These activities also put the female nurses in close proximity to the patients, stretching across the beds or with their arms wrapped round the young men to support them. Many romances started here, but not if the sister could help it.

13 Commonwealth Sisters

The thing to say at my funeral is that I always hated, loathed and despised prejudice.
Sister Joan Jenkins on return from a posting to India, 1946

By the end of the nineteenth century working overseas was becoming popular among women. They were broadening their horizons and breaking away from the Victorian restrictions of home life. They wanted more independence and adventure, and nursing provided the ideal means to achieve this ambition. There were many organizations ready to help young women to work abroad, among them the Emigration Department of the Girls' Friendly Society, the Church Societies and the Women's Emigration Society. The Agent-General in London processed the applications. These British nurses went to South Africa, America, Australia and India.

In South Africa, Sister Mary Agatha, a British-trained nurse, headed the nursing team at the New Somerset Hospital, Cape Town. The Kimberley Hospital had a large training school for nurses, where Sister Henrietta was superintendent and the Bloemfontein Sisters ran the wards. The training was aimed at refined and educated young ladies, as native servants carried out the menial work. Nurses at the Kimberley Hospital could regularly enhance their pay with private nursing for wealthy landowners.

In America all the major cities provided both training and opportunities for trained nurses. An English nurse could not have done better than head for the Philadelphia Hospital. Until 1888 a remarkable Nightingale-trained nurse, Miss Alice Fisher, held the position of Nurse Superintendent. With characteristic zeal she set about transforming this backward institution into an outstanding hospital. The authorities readily acknowledged that her dedication to improving the hospital possibly shortened her life. Such was her attachment that following her death she continued her benevolent supervision from the Woodlands Cemetery overlooking her beloved hospital, where she is forever acknowledged for her devotion to nursing.

The Bellevue Hospital, New York, prided itself on modelling its training on the principles of the Nightingale School. Sister Helen of King's College Hospital, London, headed the school. British nurses were accepted throughout America in great numbers. Hospitals in Chicago, Pennsylvania, Massachusetts and San Francisco all welcomed them. However, unlike South Africa, the plethora of British nurses meant competition for jobs and sometimes unemployment.

The Colonial Emigration Society in London reported that trained nurses who emigrated to Australia were finding great success there. Many were immediately appointed sisters or matrons of small hospitals 'up country', where new towns were forming. These hospitals followed the lead of Miss Lucy Osburn. She pioneered and transformed the struggling Sydney Royal Infirmary and introduced the Nightingale model of training throughout Australia. The Alfred Hospital, Melbourne, the General Hospital, Brisbane, and Adelaide Hospital all offered opportunities for trained nurses, although they normally trained Australian ladies. In Tasmania there were two training schools, the Hobart Hospital and Launceston General Hospital. Miss Harriet Munro, a St Bartholomew's nurse, headed the Hobart Hospital and Miss Milne from the Edinburgh Royal Infirmary, the Launceston one. Nurses were warned, however, not to consider emigrating to Australia unless they were prepared to accept the more rugged, pioneering conditions associated with the country at that time.

Nurses who went to India took short-term contracts with the Indian Nursing Service or the Lady Roberts Fund. The Indian Office in London accepted applications from candidates aged twenty-five years or over. They had to submit a recommendation from a lady in a high social position as to their suitability to join a service composed of ladies of good families. A reasonable salary, free accommodation, fuel, light and 'punkah-pullers' (men who operated the fans) awaited them.

A letter printed in *The Hospital Magazine* of 21 November 1891 offered practical advice to any nurse desirous of nursing in India. It centred on the large amount of baggage a nurse would be required to take with her. She was advised to have tin trunks principally, and one large wooden tin-lined one. It would appear that a further four large trunks would suffice, plus a good-sized cabin trunk and large Gladstone bag for cabin use. She was advised not to bring her own bath, as one would be supplied. Beds were also provided but linen had to be brought. Among many other items were 50 yards of art muslin (for curtains), gloves in a glass bottle, an imitation astrakhan coat and a riding skirt. There were about fifty sisters working in hospitals in India in 1890.

In Bombay there were three hospitals: the Benares Hospital, nursed entirely by British nurses; the Jamseeji Hospital, managed by the All Saints' Sisters; and the Cama Hospital. There were also hospitals in Madras, Calcutta and Karachi among many others. Much work however was done in smaller hospitals outside the major cities, with army officers suffering from typhoid fever, accidents or convalescing. Although a fee was charged, the British government supported these hospitals.

In the 1940s and 1950s many nurses were among the thousands of people who emigrated to Australia on assisted passage. In 1948 a friend asked Billie Cullen (née Bisland), who had trained at the Evelina Hospital for Sick Children, London, if she could leave England within two weeks; there was a post for a nursing sister on the Orient Line sailing between England and Australia. She went to another friend who had been a patient on her ward, and who was married to a vice-admiral, for advice. He asked if she really wanted the job and when she said yes, he said, 'Leave it to me.' Within days she was asked for an interview. She was very surprised to receive red carpet treatment, and was almost catapulted into the post. On board ship it was hard work, with only two sisters, two doctors and a pharmacist. On one voyage there was a flu epidemic, but they lost just one patient. Her theatre skills were used regularly, with burst gastric ulcers, and emergency appendectomies among many other ailments.

On one of these trips the boat had just left Australia when Billie was called to a young girl who had severe stomach cramps. She called the doctor, who suggested that the young lady was just about to produce a baby. Her family had emigrated to Australia on an assisted passage but the daughter was being returned to England so that the boyfriend could take responsibility for his actions. The parents had omitted to provide this information when they booked the girl's trip. The baby was born and there was a christening on board. Loaded down with a new baby and a bundle of clothing knitted by the women on board, the young lady was met by her boyfriend. Billie hoped it was a romantic and successful reunion, particularly as she had found romance of her own. On this trip she met her future husband. She had been moved to an upgraded cabin near the purser's office and was on duty while the other sister was on shore leave when the ship docked at Colombo. It was very hot, so she took iced drinks to the purser's cabin and there was Pip Cullen, the assistant purser. Neither dared let anyone know when they got engaged, or Billie would have been dismissed; they married in 1951.

Following her nurse training, Sylvia Kemp applied for work in America. Along with a friend she went to Santa Monica, California, and started nursing at St John's Hospital. Run entirely by nuns, it seemed to her more like a hotel than a hospital. After a brief interview with Sister Mary Trinatus she was employed immediately. Sylvia found it a great culture shock. The system was very relaxed, and first names were used. Soon nicknamed 'the Duchess', it took her some time to acknowledge the staff were teasing her; they were not used to her English ways. Initially she was licensed in America, not registered, so she was not allowed to work in the premature unit, which greatly interested her. She would watch what was going on through the window. This upset one doctor, who wanted to know why she was constantly watching what he was doing. Sylvia recalls, 'He nearly had me removed from the unit until it was pointed out that I was only interested in his work, so he suggested that I be allowed time to work there. They encouraged initiative!' At the hospital she found that the nursing sisters were very considerate to the nurses, and even without being asked always ensured that Sylvia and her friend had time off together. One irritation for her, however, was that she could do nothing without writing it down, otherwise there were issues of litigation. Also doctors did their own wound dressings because these were added to the patient's bill.

Jean Holland also found nursing in America different, but felt that the nurses were far more respected by the doctors. The head nurse ran the ward and first names were often used – something British nurses had difficulty with.

Wendy Carson trained at the Royal Free Hospital, London, and emigrated to Canada. She found adapting to both a small town and small hospital difficult. There was a school of nursing but it took only a short time for her to realize that they tended to treat those from outside the town as 'foreigners' – let alone those from other countries.

I decided early that I had to adopt a more Canadian accent in order to be understood by the patients following this conversation with a six-year-old boy.

Boy: How come you talk English so funny?
Me: I'm from England.
Boy: How long have you been here?
Me: Just a few weeks.
Boy: You sure learned English fast.
Me: But in England we speak English.
Boy: Well how come you talk it so funny?

Several years later when she was head nurse of a paediatric ward she had a five-year-old admitted who had only arrived three days before from his native Scotland. Most of the staff had trouble understanding him. He was shy and frightened and the staff became frustrated because he was becoming withdrawn. She had to explain to them that he was probably having as much problem understanding them as they were understanding him, and that he was refusing many things because he did not understand what they were saying.

One nurse complained to me that when she had asked the boy if he would like a popsicle and some pop, he refused. I took her back to the boy and asked him if her would like an ice lolly and some lemonade and was greeted with a broad grin and 'Yes please!' I then sat down and made a list of things for the staff, with everyday words they could use that the boy would understand. So it became a two-way learning process and in the end all were happy.

172

On arrival in Canada Wendy discovered that her nursing experience in England counted for little. Working on a paediatric unit she had to watch a demonstration on how to bath a baby, and then bath one under supervision. In England she had been teaching mothers how to wash babies in a parentcraft unit for six months. Medical terminologies were also often different, and medications were known by their manufacturers' names. Babies' feeds would come direct from a diet kitchen, with nothing readily available for new admissions. Snacks for older children were sent from the kitchen on a regular basis, but they were always what the dietitians thought the children wanted, and there was no flexibility on the ward for any alternative.

Rosemary James, who now lives in America, completed her nurse training before moving to Canada. She felt that she had been well prepared for any move abroad with a clinical tutor who included in their training such things as cupping, an archaic treatment even in the 1940s. This entailed the use of a cupping glass that was heated so that the air was removed to cause suction. It was placed over the skin to draw blood o the surface for slow blood-letting. When her students looked somewhat puzzled, the tutor told them, 'You will not all go on to work in modern hospitals; some of you could be working in Africa or India, then you will need to know such things.' For Rosemary it was to be the prairies of Canada. Here the hospital was small and had previously been a bank. There were just three nursing sisters, one for each shift, and a doctor who served a 60-mile radius. She was informed that if she had a patient with a 'hot' appendix she was to place an icebag over the site until the doctor's return. When it came to her first surgery case she was handed a bottle of ether and told to keep the patient's chin up and drip the ether slowly over a mask. The patient was to undergo a vaginal hysterectomy. Extremely anxious she ensured that she very firmly held the patient's jaw up throughout the operation. For some time after, the patient complained that her jaw and neck ached, and she could not understand why. It was much later that Rosemary explained what had happened and by then they had become good friends. 'I think the other big shock in Canada was when we were told not to do anything with a dead patient, just call the funeral home. My first patient died sitting in a chair and there he stayed all night until the funeral people arrived.'

Like many nurses Audrey Jones had a sense of adventure and an urge to travel.

When travelling abroad in the 1940s, distances were not as we know them now, Even France seemed such a long way off. My journey to Africa took three weeks by ship, then a three-day train journey. I started on a ward but as soon as they realized I was theatre trained, into the theatre I went.

Having had experience in thoracic surgery she was expected to take over a theatre for heart surgery.

No one else had this experience and so I was considered very useful. I was thrown in and how I was thrown in. I worked with a Professor Fatti and Mr Whitehead, who were pioneering heart surgery at that time. Blaylock's operation for mitral stenosis was quite new in the fifties. It was a steep learning curve.

All the sisters were English and the attendants mostly Afrikaans. The cleaners were black Africans. It was a constant job keeping order as the Afrikaans people would not speak English. 'You got by but you were made fully aware that you were resented, but they were very hard working.' The hospital could not keep the African 'lads' for long as they were mainly working in the hospital to earn a dowry.

They seemed more interested in being able to buy a cow. If you wanted them to collect something from another hospital you had to tell them it was needed immediately or you might not see them for the rest of that day. They were so easily distracted. When they met friends they just wanted a chat, they were so friendly. You quickly learned that you could not put different tribes together because of tribal disharmony. You soon got used to it but it was a real eye opener.

Audrey also found that there was a large Jewish community, so there were many circumcisions. The chief rabbi was not very skilled, so the family would also pay for a surgeon and sister to stand by to repair any damage.

I felt so sorry, these poor boys would bleed dreadfully. Initially we did not realize that when a boy was circumcized it was a very important event. On the office desk we found these beautiful biscuits and a bottle of wine; thinking it was for us sisters we ate the biscuits and drank the wine. When the patient came out he looked longingly for the wine and biscuits, which he certainly had earned, and we had to make excuses. It was all part of learning when you worked abroad.

Later she worked at the Groote Schuur Hospital in Cape Town, where Christiaan Barnard pioneered the first heart transplant surgery in 1967.

Margaret Watts, who trained at Farnborough Hospital went to South Africa in the 1950s, thinking that apartheid might not be as strict as it was portrayed in the media. It was, but she soon learned that as an individual there was little that she could do about it. First she travelled to Port Shepstone on the Natal south coast to nurse with the Natal Provincial Administration. It was here that she realized that British-trained nurses had a broader range of nursing skills; by not specializing too early they adapted to different types of nursing.

From there she went to King Edward VIII Hospital, Congella, Durban, to work with African and Indian patients. Here she was sister of the children's medical ward. The wards had about sixty beds, thirty each side. On the floor at either side of each bed were mattresses with more patients on. So where there was a bed 1, there would also be beds 1a and 1b, and at very busy times even a bed 1c. This meant that there could be 120 patients at a time, prompting the classic exchange, 'Sister, do you mean the patient on the bed or the one on the mattress?' 'No, Doctor, I mean the patient on the chair!' On intake day between thirty-two and thirty-four very ill patients would be admitted, some who had walked up to 40 miles to the hospital. 'As ward sister,' recalls Margaret, 'I would go round to see who the doctors had to visit, particularly those who would not have survived that night. Initially it was very different, but this was a training hospital with high standards, so I soon adapted.' Here the sisters had to do a spell of night duty, responsible for six to eight wards, many with over 100 patients. It took a long time to get round two visits a night; security staff escorted them the whole time.

Witch doctors were traditionally very influential, and they were wary of what was going on in the hospitals.

One of the doctors pointed out to me that on the veranda a patient was being visited by one of these witch doctors. We went out to see what was going on and the doctor said, 'Let's take a picture of you with him; if he agrees I will give him some olive oil as a present,' which we did.

He told the doctor, who could speak Zulu, that he was going round looking at his defectors who had gone over to European medicine, 'but he was probably trying to make sure that they came back to him afterwards,' said Margaret.

She then proceeded north to Zululand. Being the only one with the necessary experience, apart from the matron, she immediately took charge of the operating theatre because of a shortage. Here the staff consisted solely of Dick, a local Zulu. What she could not do he could, and they ran the place between them. There would be the major cases in the morning, and with the surgeon they would just manage. After an operation Dick would clean and scrub the instruments, Margaret would check them over, prepare the instruments for the next operation and pack the drums for sterilization.

There was a very easy relationship with the doctors and surgeons in small hospitals of about two hundred beds, so of course we were all able to interact together. It was hard work; after a full day's list the theatre would be readied for any emergencies. When I had the time I would be off to the golf course to knock a few balls around, if there was a problem back I would go; all very casual considering what I had been used to.

Audrey Phillips applied to Canada to nurse in 1965. She applied through Canada House and thought she had the offer of a job in the Holy Cross Hospital in Vancouver. When she got there she contacted the hospital, only to be told that they were not expecting her and there were no vacancies. Fortunately she had a friend she could stay with. It appears that sending nurses out to other countries with no proper job to go to was not unusual. Being trained at St Thomas's

Hospital, she quickly gained employment at the Vancouver General Hospital, and within two weeks was promoted to head nurse. This quick promotion she knows upset many of the other nurses.

Another cautionary tale comes from Betty Blacklar, who trained at Radcliffe Hospital. Following her brother to Kenya at the end of the Second World War, she was to look after both the first and the second child his wife was expecting. She did, however, demand that a return ticket be provided if the arrangement did not work out. She liked Kenya and as well as looking after the children she had several other jobs, one of which was looking after a man with a crushed leg; his wife had run over him with a combine harvester. She refused to allow the doctors to amputate the leg and decided to take him to England for a second opinion, taking Betty with her. Six seats were removed from the cabin of the Constellation to accommodate him; the flight took two days. On landing in England they went to the Seaman's Hospital, Albert Docks, where they knew an administrator. The matron was not happy about having a 'private' sister on her ward but relented and provided a sister's bedroom attached to the ward. This meant that Betty would be on twenty-four-hour call. Following remedial surgery to the leg, at which the surgeon demanded Betty's attendance, the wife had her husband removed to a guesthouse in the New Forest. Here things got a little out of hand, with the wife spending more and more time away from the house with a series of suitors. It could not last, 'The final straw came,' Betty said, 'when one of these suitors left his two young children for me to look after as well as the husband. It happened to be the point I also realized that all was not in order financially.' She demanded a flight back to Kenya, which was provided but a bill for her time was completely ignored. Later she found out that the surgeon's bill was also ignored, and the bill for the three months' accommodation in the New Forrest.

The flow was not all one way. A great contribution came to British hospitals from overseas. In the late 1960s the British government encouraged people from the Commonwealth countries to come to Britain because of shortages of labour, particularly in the public services and health.

Lynette Patterson (née Small) arrived in England on 21 March 1958 from Guyana to pursue a nursing course at the Manor Hospital, Epsom, a hospital for the mentally deficient (now known as learning difficulties). She thought she was applying to be trained as a nurse in acute mental illness, but after her initial disappointment she took wholeheartedly to this field, finding the work both rewarding and inspiring. She was warmly welcomed by the matron and staff, who made her feel not only at home but valued and cared for. Throughout her training she was respected and at no time felt discriminated against. But she still wanted to achieve her ambition to work with the mentally ill. She spent two years training at Long Grove Hospital, then had to break to have her family and she was unable to take her final examination. Returning to nursing in 1964 she chose to work with mentally handicapped children at the Queen Mary's Hospital for Children, London. After working there for six months the matron suggested she apply for the post of sister on a specialist ward for autistic and psychotic children. Because of the speciality she had many student nurses working on the ward from psychiatry and general nursing. This encouraged her in two directions. First she gained her general nurse certificate and then decided that she should work towards a qualification in education, the Clinical Teacher Certificate. In 1972 she was invited by the matron to transfer to the school to do full-time teaching. In this post she became the only female black teacher in the mental handicap sector. To further her teaching skills she took a postgraduate Bachelor of Arts course in the education of adults.

Dorothy Turner trained at Bolingbroke Hospital, Clapham, from 1962 to 1965. At the age of twenty it was a great shock coming from Jamaica, to find England so cold. The winter of 1962 was the worst for years. 'One day the heavens opened and the roads froze. I had never seen the likes of it before, so I wrote to my mother and said, you will never believe it, we are walking on ice.' Dorothy had always wanted to be a midwife, and applied from Jamaica to train as one only to find that she could only become a midwife if she first trained as a general nurse. The main reason why she applied to Bolingbroke Hospital was because she had a brother living there.

In 1962, we were very naive young girls and certainly the set I joined was. I also think that when I started nursing and certainly among the group I was with we still wanted to nurse the patient, money hardly came into it. Of that group five of us became great friends, we were a mixture of Jamaican, Barbadian, Spanish and African.

Training at Bolingbroke Hospital Dorothy became lifelong friends with Cynthia Braithwaite from Barbados. Cynthia spent most of her nursing career at Bolingbroke, 'where we all studied together, laughed together, cried together and passed together'. Dorothy and Cynthia also went out for evenings together. On one occasion they were on a late-night pass to go to a dance and inevitably came back late. Having left a window open, they climbed into the nurses' home, only to be met by the night sister, who fortunately found it most amusing and did not report them for the matron's 'parade' in the morning. Cynthia was the sister of the out-patient and casualty departments. Here she had departments for eye care, geriatrics, psychiatry, rheumatology, fracture and urology. She soon learned that when a patient said, 'Can you hurry sister? I have left some potatoes on the boil', there was little danger of them boiling over; it was one among many excuses that were used to get an early appointment.

Dorothy's original intention had been to do only midwifery but she enjoyed almost every minute of her nurse training and would not have missed it for the world. She cannot speak too highly of Matron Annie Lane. 'I can't ever forget her, she was wonderful. Because so many of us were from overseas she was very protective, and she knew each of our names, which was remarkable considering the numbers involved.' Dorothy remembers her saying, 'You must feed yourselves, nursing is hard work you know! I know I am not your mother but you are a long way from home and so I need to be here to mother you.' She would also say to the nurses, 'Always think of yourself in that bed and then work out how you would like to be treated.'

In 1966 Dorothy applied to work on a gynaecology ward at a hospital in London. 'Here for the first time I was faced with terminations. This proved very difficult for me because of personal and religious convictions. After a short time it created a huge dilemma for me. On one occasion I had to provide a dish for one of these terminations and the foetus was twenty weeks old.' It was at this hospital that she first met racism. The white nurses all sat at the front of the classroom and the non-whites sat at the back. 'When I enquired into this I was told this had always been the case. I left after only three months.'

179

From this experience she decided to follow her first desire and started her midwifery training at Redhill Hospital and her part two at Beckenham Hospital. After promotion to sister in 1970 she again found some discrimination.

I was on night duty when this young girl was brought in; the mother did not know she was pregnant, neither did her father until he had to bring her to the maternity department. By now she was well into her labour. He rang the bell and when they entered he immediately announced that he did not want a black nurse attending to his daughter. I told him there were only black nurses. I was not prepared to argue any more and took over by concentrating on the mother.

Dorothy took her upstairs to the ward and was immediately called back as the father had collapsed with a heart attack. 'So I ended up caring for him as well until the ambulance came. I don't think it would have changed his mind! Apparently people like him don't mess about, they just tell you straight out, but I must say apart from these incidents I have met little if any other prejudice.' Because of the changes taking place in the health service and particularly education Dorothy reluctantly took early retirement. It was not that she could not accept change; as she said, 'In order to grow and develop there has to be change.' But having enjoyed non-discriminatory practices in her nursing career she was not prepared to risk facing possible discrimination as nurse education became first college then university based.

Janet Campbell left her home country of Guyana in 1965. Her father was a teacher so her intention was to follow him into school, but as a school health nurse. To achieve this ambition she had to train as a nurse. Her application for training was sent directly to the Ministry of Health as no one could apply straight to a hospital from abroad. When the ministry had accepted her application, then she could apply to hospitals. She deliberately chose Loughborough as she wanted to be in the countryside rather than in a major city. She found the town, though not the weather, similar in a way to Guyana, in that it was small at that time and everyone knew everyone else. When she arrived the Mayor gave a big reception for all the overseas students.

'It was the same at Christmas,' she remembers. 'They always made us feel as though we belonged. You would be put with a local family and on Christmas Day be invited for dinner. So that on Christmas Day even though I desperately wanted to be with my own family there was no reason to feel alone.'

Janet had intended to do her general training but the bed numbers at the hospital had been reduced by the time she started, and it became an enrolled training hospital. On completing her enrolled training she was encouraged by the tutor, Miss Fulton, to do her general training. 'When I went to do my training the tutor openly resented nurses who had been through enrolled training. No matter how well we did she always managed to make us feel inferior.' After nevertheless successfully completing her training she moved to the South-western General Hospital, London.

It was noticed that I was particularly good with the elderly. This did not make much sense to me because I just treated them as I would my own parents. It was not till later that I became aware that nurses tended to avoid working in this area. Matron in particular pointed this out to me; this is what enthused me to work with the elderly, and so I became a specialist in this care.

She was promoted to sister on an elderly care ward. 'I found the role of sister a mixture of being efficient, the work had to be done, and at the same time giving time to the patients and staff. I always avoided telling staff off; I found other ways round problems if I could.' She would do her ward round and note any problems the patients had.

I would then say to the nurse, when they had finished their work to always go round and check. Then they could either give themselves a pat on the back by admiring what they had done or change anything that needed to be changed. Then I would check when she was on again, go round her patients and then find her and praise her work. It is far better than telling a nurse off.

A devout Christian from a traditionally religious family – her father retired from teaching and became a priest – it was always important

181

for Janet to meet the spiritual needs of patients, without preaching in any way to them. 'It was the time when we were breaking away from the stigma of geriatric care and moving towards person-centred care'.

Jean Bajnath (née Hussain) felt she wanted to travel and experience a different life. Life in Guyana for a young woman was very restrictive, being chaperoned everywhere by a parent or brother. 'It was nice not having these restrictions,' she said. 'I did not like the weather; it was so very cold, and it was a shock to see trees without leaves on, they looked to me like dead twigs. I had never seen that before; where I came from the trees were always green.' She pointed out that in Guyana it was a tradition for everyone to own his or her own home, even if it was a shack, and also for everyone to work. If someone could not get paid work then they would have to be self-sufficient. So when she arrived in England the first two issues were to get a job and accommodation.

Nursing solved both these problems for me. It was also agreeable to my parents, as there was the matron who was responsible for me like a parent. And there were other people who you could socialize and talk with; you were not isolated. The hospital system was very strict but that suited me, my home life had been strict.

Jean was accepted for thoracic nurse training at Milford Chest Hospital, Surrey, having no idea what she was applying for apart from wanting to train as a nurse. 'To be honest I felt I was more a part of the domestic staff than nursing. I spent most of my time in the sluice area polishing metal bedpans and sputum mugs with methylated spirit. Every bit of clothing and linen was sluiced before it went to the laundry. It was a cleaning job.'

Clarence Bajnath came to England from Trinidad to further his education.

When I came to England my intention was to enter medicine. I was working for the High Commission in the West Indian Federation Department, Burton Street, London. In this post we dealt with a lot of students coming into the country. From this experience I looked at nursing as a possible route into medicine. Not quite sure where I wanted to go, I certainly did not want to move further north, as I was still adjusting to the cold weather, and I did not want to stay in London, it was too crowded. So I applied and was accepted at Milford Hospital, Surrey, to train for the British Thoracic Nursing Certificate.

So Jean Hussain and Clarence Bajnath met at Milford Hospital during their training in thoracic nursing. Clarence recalled:

We married in 1963. We both lived in nursing homes at the hospital, separate male and female of course. We decided to get married in a registrar's office, mainly to keep it quiet. We were able to live in our individual rooms for a while with Jean wearing her ring only when we were out together. The two of us were very naive and thought we could get away with it.

It did not take long before others got to hear of their marriage.

We were immediately hauled before matron in her office. She said, 'What did you think you were doing? I could sack you both for this.' When she calmed down she congratulated us but of course we then had to find accommodation outside the hospital. We had a son a year later so it meant I really had to buckle down and concentrate on a career in nursing.

Following this training there was a joint decision to move to Portsmouth to do their general nurse training.

In the last forty years there has been a massive increase in overseas personnel from all parts of the world. Without this highly valued resource the National Health Service as we know it would not have survived. Margaret Brayton was the Executive Secretary of the Commonwealth Nurses' Federation from its foundation in 1973 to her retirement in 1993. Under her guidance regional networks of nursing associations were set up to campaign for the establishment of colleges of nursing in West Africa, the South Pacific and the Caribbean. These have now developed their own courses of study and textbooks. Her contribution to Commonwealth nursing and the pioneering activities she promoted were recognized in 1989 with the award of the MBE.

Roy Stallard recently visited South Africa, where he found their hospitals successfully maintaining the traditional role of matron. Matron Smit continues her regular wards rounds at the Parowmedica Clinic, Cape Town, and as Roy said, 'They also continue with the traditional ward sister!'

14   Military Sisters

Nursing Sisters: Arrangements have been made for a limited number of Nursing Sisters to be trained in military hospitals under the auspices of the National Society of Aid to the Sick and Wounded in War . . . Preference will be given to widows and daughters of military officers.

Notice in *The Times* and *Daily Telegraph*, 1881

Nursing is steeped in military history. Unlike the early sisterhoods, however, military nursing took decades to become respected. Women as nurses were scarcely mentioned in early military histories, but there are indications that as early as the Roman period they were involved in nursing, and they were allowed to join the crusaders of the Order of the Knights of St John in Palestine. In 1690 the first army staff hospitals appeared. These were either fixed hospitals that later developed into general hospitals, or mobile hospitals that developed into flying hospitals. The flying hospitals were noted for their camp followers, ladies who were either the wives of serving men or ladies of ill-repute, and when necessary they could be employed to nurse the sick and wounded. Donald Munroe, physician to George III's army, championed the cause of women in military hospitals and by the end of the eighteenth century a female nurse's pay was one shilling a day, a not inconsiderable sum for that time. In the *Gentleman's Magazine* of 1746, there was an extract from a marine's diary which said, 'A great number of women have enlisted on board the fleet (Portsmouth) bound for Cape Breton, and continue to enter daily. They are allowed ten pounds each and their provisions during the passage, and when they arrive are to receive further encouragement.' This marine would not have been surprised by this activity, as

185

women on board ships were not new. They were paid for laundering and for nursing the sick and injured.

There were few fixed military hospitals before the nineteenth century but women were regularly employed in those that existed until 1832. They were then discouraged until later in the century. By then it was common and legitimate practice for women to follow the army on campaigns, nursing the sick and wounded. One of these women, Mrs George (Annie) Fox, proved so outstanding in attending the wounded under fire in the first Boer War 1880–1 that she was the first woman to be honoured with a full military funeral. Women of course were prominent in the Crimean War, but it was not until 1866 that a royal warrant was issued authorizing the appointment of nursing sisters in any military general hospitals. That same year Mrs Shaw Stuart became Superintendent at the Herbert (Military) Hospital at Woolwich. Three years later Jane Deeble went from St Thomas's Hospital, London, to be Superintendent at the Royal Victoria Hospital, Netley. She was a widow; her husband, Surgeon-Major John Deeble, was killed in the Abyssinian campaign. After some time in the Zulu Wars she was appointed the first Superintendent of the Army Nursing Service in 1881. Not content with this, she and twenty-four nurses went off to the Egyptian Campaign in 1882. She retired in 1890; Miss H. Campbell Norman was appointed Superintendent the same year.

The headquarters for naval nursing was Haslar Hospital, Gosport, where in 1884 the authorities realized the necessity for improving the standard of nursing care. They established a group of trained sick-berth attendants, and in the same year appointed a small staff of well-educated female nurses with a head sister, Louisa Hogg. The medical officers received the first group with delight – they were men – and the second with some animosity – they were women. In the wards the nurses were addressed as 'madam' by staff and patients. Being trained nurses they were responsible for the practical instruction of the newly formed sick-berth attendants. They quickly established themselves and soon became highly respected by the medical staff.

Florence Nightingale had wanted to limit women's involvement in military hospitals because of a concern that they might make life too easy for servicemen. She thought that over-indulgence and too much comfort would encourage the men to stay in hospital, and that a military hospital should remain different from a civilian establishment, both in discipline and in detail, altogether a 'rougher and ruder' place. The nurses were often reduced to doing little more than fanning patients or placing ice in their mouths when they were in a fever, and helping them to be more comfortable in bed. They were not able to wash more than a 'discreet' part of the servicemen, nor were they permitted to change their dressings. Where the female nurses in civilian hospitals were taking more responsibility for this work, in military hospitals it took much longer for them to be accepted by the medical staff.

To be eligible to join the army or naval nursing service, a woman was expected to provide evidence that she had completed three years' training in a good general hospital. She also had to produce a recommendation from a person of standing to the effect that she possessed the right personal qualities for the post. A sister would start on a salary of £30 per year in 1880.

Men were excluded from training in civilian hospitals but offered training in both the army and navy hospitals. Therefore the only way for men to enter general nurse training was to enlist as a soldier or sailor. The term of enlistment for military nursing was seven years, plus five years on the reserve. Training was available at the military hospitals in all branches of nursing, under the direction of the matrons and sisters of the Queen Alexandra's Imperial Military Nursing Service (QAIMNS). Applicants had to be between eighteen and twenty-five and at least 5 feet 3 inches tall. No previous knowledge of nursing or medicine was required, although an ability to write a short composition and do simple arithmetic was essential.

Initial training included instruction in drill and the techniques of stretcher drill, ambulance work and first aid. They were then deemed to be ready for ward work in the hospitals. After a year of instruction and practical ward work under sisters, they had an examination in elementary nursing, anatomy and physiology. If they passed they became class III nursing orderlies. Those who showed special aptitude for nursing and gained the appropriate educational levels were able to go on to become class I nursing orderlies. These qualifications were not recognized by civilian nursing authorities. Other opportunities were open to men in radiography, dispensary, massage and mental illness. After three full years' training a few of these men who had shown exemplary skill and educational ability could be admitted to the QAIMNS.

For those who chose nursing in the navy the rules were slightly different. Here they were known as sick-berth attendants, and had to sign on for twelve years' continuous service. They had to be between eighteen and twenty-two and at least 5 feet 4 inches tall; those accepted entered as probationary sick-berth attendants. The probationers were employed in the royal naval hospitals, harbour ships, and sea-going ships. Following successful training they would be promoted to second sick-birth attendant then through to chief sick-berth attendant. They were paid more for working in zymotic (infectious diseases) or lunatic wards. The highest promotion for these attendants was head wardmaster at the naval hospitals of Chatham, Haslar, Plymouth, Portland, Malta and Gibraltar, and in two hospital ships.

Before the Second World War, military hospital accommodation comprised approximately 9,000 beds, of which 2,000 were in use. By the end of the war, the number of occupied beds had increased to over 350,000. This expansion was brought about by using existing military hospitals, new military hospitals, beds in general hospitals, mental hospitals, poor law institutions, and territorial force general hospitals. The three largest military hospitals before the war were the Royal Victoria Hospital, Netley, with 955 beds, the Herbert Hospital, Woolwich, with over 600 beds, and the Connaught Hospital, Aldershot, with nearly 500.

With the desire for nurses to travel abroad, increasing numbers joined the Queen Alexandra's Royal Army Nursing Corps (QARANC), formerly the QAIMNS, the Queen Alexandra's Royal Naval Nursing Service (QARNNS), or the Princess Mary's Royal Air Force Nursing Service (PMRAFNS) formerly, the Royal Air Force Nursing Service. Many of the new recruits on short-term commissions were very disappointed to find that they were not being offered overseas postings. On extending their commission, however, they nearly always found they were posted overseas and many could spend much of their time abroad.

Towards the end of the Second World War a telegram came to Joan Jennings who was in the QAIMNS reserves, requesting her to report at once for immediate military nursing service in Palestine. She sailed out on the *Empress of Britain* and was surprised to find that her destination was in fact to be India. She was immediately shocked at the snobbery.

> The first thing my bearer said to me was, 'Can I get you a better napkin ring?' The sisters all had finger bowls and they never picked up a tennis ball and never carried water, a boy carried the water. I had a nice hut; at the back of the hut was a tin bath and commode that within moments of being used the sweeper emptied. The sweeper squatted out all day waiting for someone to use the commode.

The sisters could only go to the first house cinema if they were in evening dress. 'And there was a war on, would you believe it?'

The matron put Joan in charge of the prisoner-of-war hospital. Every night a bearer would go in front of her and hit the grass to scare away the snakes. She would enter a large concrete building where there were two Anglo-Indian warders and the rest of the helpers were Italians, called *infameros*. The doctors were all prisoners of war. An officer's wife had heard one of them playing the piano in Rome before the war – he was a concert pianist – and she sent her own grand piano so that he could continue to play.

> He would come and check with me on what drugs were wanted, and then he would say, 'What would you like to hear tonight sister', and I would say Chopin or Tchaikovsky and he would play just for me. In the prison hospital the prisoners and nurses had great fun. They used to say *finito* Churchill, and I would say *finito* Mussolini and they would roar with laughter. Germans and Tommies could be on the same ward and they would exchange cigarettes. The thing to say at my funeral is that I always hated, loathed and despised prejudice.

There are endless stories of quiet heroism among military sisters in wartime. Just one example was that of Julie Gillespie whose actions were reported in the *Sunday Pictorial* of 27 August 1944. The reporter stood in the hold of the cross-Channel steamer carrying wounded soldiers back from Normandy. He watched as the surgeon opened a man's leg, exposing the splintered bone. On the other side of the makeshift operating table stood Julie Gillespie. Her hair was tucked in a skull-cap and her mouth covered by a pad; only her eyes were visible and she did not even blink when a mine exploded. 'It was as if a giant hand had slapped the side of the boat,' he reported, and Julie and the surgeon just carried on. Julie was one of five sisters aboard this Red Cross carrier who had all been with the boat since its first trip, on D-Day-plus-two, when they collected the initial wounded. This was their thirty-fourth trip across these mine-infested waters.

Julie had started her nursing career at the age of seventeen in Glasgow and volunteered for the Territorial Army Nursing Service at the outbreak of war. Some of the 6,000 servicemen who were evacuated on her ship did not survive the trip back to England and Julie held the hand of many a soldier as he died on board. As they landed and the wounded were evacuated ashore, the reporter's last sight of her was as she stood on the gangplank waving. She then turned back into the ship. With her charges safely landed there was much to do to ready the steamer for its next crossing.

There is also a military role in times of peace. Joan Pease trained at East Surrey Hospital, Redhill, in 1946. Following midwifery training and experience as a ward sister she decided to join the army. She recognizes that this must have been a major decision, but she says:

> I really do not know why. I should give some grand reason. I have even asked my friends to try and work out when and how it came about. I simply wrote off to the Ministry of Defence and was given an interview and accepted as a lieutenant in QARANC. I suppose one incentive but not a reason, was that in Nottingham I was on a salary of £20 a month, and when I joined the army I got 15s 6p (77½p) a day.

Joan found the interview both challenging and interesting, especially when she was asked if she could play bridge or ride: 'It was all very social,' she remarked. 'I also had a surprise when the sister who took me for my medical was wearing lipstick, a thing I had never seen before in a hospital.' Something else she found unusual was calling people by their Christian name. 'Never would we have done that in a civilian hospital. This included the matron when we were off duty.' The challenge came from learning a different way of life, a military way, but although it was markedly more disciplined it was less authoritarian than her experience in civilian hospitals. 'It was strict, yes,' she said, 'but my generation did not mind that, we were brought up with it in our families. At the same time there was also a unique sense of freedom which we all enjoyed.'

In May 1953, Joan started a basic training course at Liphook, Hampshire. Her first overseas posting was to Egypt in 1956, the year of the Suez crisis, and from there she was sent to the British military hospital, Nicosia, Cyprus. In 1955 a Greek Cypriot organization, EOKA, led by Archbishop Makarios and General Grivas, had begun guerrilla warfare against the British. These two postings gave Joan her first experience in gunshot and blast injuries, experience she would take to a wing of Musgrave Park Hospital, Belfast, from 1973 to 1974.

It was an extraordinarily good life; hard work, yes, but also we had our social life laid on for us. For instance when I first went to dinner in the mess the matron said, 'Come and sit by me, Miss Pease.' I had to sit there and was expected to make conversation. This way it was thought you learned how to make polite talk, and how to mix at dinner. It was very important in those days.

Joan gradually moved up the promotion ladder and was promoted to major, where she still had contact with the wards and patients.

Later in her career when she was Deputy Commodore at the QARANC depot and training establishment at Hindhead, she asked the new recruits what bothered them the most. 'I was surprised to be told that it was not the basic discipline but learning to use the cutlery on a laid-up dinner table. I guess it will be even worse now that so much food is eaten in front of the television.' She retired as Colonel Deputy Director of Nursing Services at the Ministry of Defence.

Angela Scofield gained her state registration at University College, London, and following her midwifery part one worked at St Mary's Hospital, Bristol, a private hospital run by the Little Sisters of Christ. A year in Australia and another as a sister at Bristol Royal Infirmary made her rethink her role. She wrote down the pros and cons of staying where she was or taking a radical step into the forces. 'I had a friend I discussed this with, and he said to go for it, so I did!' At thirty she thought she might be too old, but not so; she joined the Princess Mary's Royal Air Force Nursing Service in March 1980. At this time the RAF changed its rank structure. On 31 March, her first day of service was as a flight officer. 'I was told not to get too used to it; the next day I became a flight lieutenant. So I was the last flight officer to be commissioned in the Princess Mary's.'

Angela commenced her military nursing at RAF Hospital Wroughton on a genito-urinary ward.

> I found it strange at first. In a civilian hospital I was the only sister on a ward with staff nurses and student nurses. In the RAF I was a sister, but on the ward would be other sisters. This intriguing situation was sorted out by rank. I rather enjoyed it, it was very liberating, I really could work directly with the patients and do clinical nursing.

Following a period of service at RAF Hospital Wegberg, West Germany, Angela was promoted to Flight Nursing Officer and returned to RAF Wroughton to be part of the air medical evacuation team. There were ten sisters in the team, two of whom were male. They were responsible for collecting and bringing back to the United Kingdom servicemen, their families and embassy staff for treatment. This service worked on a priority system of one to four, depending on the severity of the case. Priority one was an emergency, priority four was someone who required a specialist out-patient appointment. The service entailed flights to Germany, Ascension Island, the Falklands, Cyprus and Hong Kong. There were other flights to all points around the world to pick up naval personnel.

Although they were sometimes known as the 'Glamour Girls', the work was often anything but glamorous. They could end up flying for hours in uncomfortable aeroplanes with few facilities.

> We would land and then have to set off again with little sleep or rest. I always had my suitcase packed. I will never forget bringing a little boy back from the Falklands; he was about

192

eight years old. We landed at Brize Norton and I have never seen that journey to Walton through such different eyes. He kept saying, 'Mummy, Mummy, there's a bus, there's a pillar box, Mummy there's a bridge.' He had only seen pictures of these things; I was astonished.

Promoted to squadron leader, Angela was moved to Headley Court, a 'tri-service' rehabilitation unit where following their initial recovery from injury servicemen were given the full benefit of medical rehabilitation. Here the patients would have a full working day organized and supervized by therapists. Angela's unit dealt specifically with head injuries. 'Some of these patients would be on my unit for months as there was much slower progress. It could be very frustrating watching a patient struggling for an age trying to put her socks on. We had speech therapists and cognitive psychologists as well as the other therapists.' It was a truly collective effort, encapsulating Headley Court's motto *Per mutua* ('by mutual effort').

Angela was chosen to lead a nursing team at RAF Hospital Muharraq, in Bahrain, at the commencement of the Gulf War. 'It was remarkable really,' she recalls, 'men being able to phone home to their wives, get an earful about the kiddies, then go to war. Pilots living in relative luxury in a hotel one minute and then having to fly incredibly difficult missions over enemy territory – and we could watch it on television.' She was chosen to lead the female flight in the Gulf War parade in London. Awarded the Associate Royal Red Cross Medal, she retired as a wing commander (matron) in 1998.

Flight Officer Mary Rose Ellis (later Wrangham) was chosen to work at RAF Halton, Aylesbury, in 1957 and allocated to the renal unit team. Part of the ward was set up for renal dialysis.

It was very Heath Robinson. The dialysis machine looked like a Bendix washing machine with a circular tube for the centrifugal area. The outer ring cleansed the fluid that had passed from the patient into the middle part then to the outer. There were tubes, monitors, drips; you name it, there was paraphernalia all over the place, there was no room to move.

Group Captain Jackson led the team and it was Mary's role to nurse the patients when the dialysis machine was in operation. Blood pressure, pulse and respiration were recorded quarter-hourly. The group captain would not allow any change-over of staff during this experimental procedure without his express permission. 'So to keep us all going,' she said, 'he generously supplied us with a bag of Fox's Glacier Mints and glasses of water, and that was it!'

In keeping with the aim of the service this team was always ready to fly anywhere by helicopter to administer urgent dialysis. The patients the team dealt with were service personnel or civilians, with a preference for those who were fit and healthy to start with.

One patient was from South Africa. He was involved in a serious car accident and the only survivor. He was a big man and his language was extremely coarse, his blaspheming in front of us was almost unbearable, it was so unusual for those days. To make things worse he was not allowed solids and craved for Pepsi Cola. He spent three months with us. His wife came to stay with him towards the end, which made him a lot better behaved.

Another patient had collapsed with kidney disease and fallen off a ladder in Blackpool. He came to visit them after he had recovered to take Mary and Group Captain Jackson out to dinner. Mary recalls, 'He called at the office to ask for me and Jacko, and off the three of us went to dinner in Wendover.' The group captain had a growing family and their joke was that their dad liked kidneys for breakfast, dinner and tea. When Mary thinks of dialysis treatment now she is very proud to have been there at the start.

At the age of twenty-five Liz Carter (née Ebdon) decided that a four-year contract with the QARNNS would be an opportunity both to expand her career and broaden her outlook. Initially she was surprised at the enormous respect she received as a QARNNS sister. 'I felt that I was treated like a princess and, as for being saluted, well!' One of her postings was to Malta where she met her future husband, Stephen, a purser supply officer. He was one of the three bachelors based there; the other two also married QARNNS sisters. They became engaged in Malta and on their return to Haslar Hospital,

Gosport, they decided to marry. Up to this time female personnel had been expected to leave when they married; Liz was the first to marry and remain in the service. She also had her first child, David, in the service. 'I tried hard to hide the bulge,' she recalls, 'and as you can guess there were some strange looks from the stuffy older hierarchy when my apron would not meet at the back and was done up with six nappy pins under my belt.' This was 1977, when commissioning was introduced in the QARNNS, so her commission was in her married name of Carter.

All three services are primarily nursing services, but each continues to have military responsibilities. Since their various beginnings, this military responsibility has taken the nurses into conflict areas around the world. In recent years they have been active in the Falklands and the Gulf. Although no women served on the Falkland Islands, QARRNS sisters were on board the SS *Uganda* receiving the injured from the conflict and QARANC sisters sailed out on the TEV *Rangatira*. Here they set up 2 Field Hospital in what had been the King Edward Memorial Hospital. More recently RFA *Argus* has been involved in the two gulf wars. The PMRAFNS were active transporting the injured from both these conflicts.

Men in the military nursing services could be married, but they could not be officers. John Greene was due to be called up for service in 1940 when he saw an advertisement for qualified mental nurses to join the navy as sick-berth attendants. Shortly after applying he received a call to report to Butlins Holiday Camp, Skegness, then known as HMS *Royal Arthur*. There he joined twenty-nine other volunteers. In their twelve weeks' training they were shown how to salute and fire a rifle. They were now members of HM Royal Naval Sick Berth Attendants (SBA). Life in the hospitals ran strictly on naval lines, similar to a ship at sea. When he was senior nurse on duty and a high-ranking male officer or the matron did an inspection he would have to remove his nurse gown, put on a cap, step forward, salute and say, 'SBA Greene, sir (or madam), twenty-eight patients all present and correct.' Every patient who was not on bed-rest, had to stand by his bed.

In 1944 he was posted to a hospital ship, the SS *Vita*, bound for Port Said on its way to the Far East. It had two large medical and surgical wards, a well-equipped operating theatre and a special ward for psychiatric patients, which was to be his unit. The staff consisted of a surgeon captain, a surgeon lieutenant, five naval sisters, a matron and a nursing staff of SBAs. The officers had separate messes, where the sisters also dined. Even as the specialist psychiatric nurse in charge of the unit, John was always subordinate to the most junior sister.

In the Far East he was constantly called on to work with traumatized servicemen who had been involved in heavy fighting. But nothing, he felt, could compare with those returning on the troop ship to England in October 1945. There were hundreds of emaciated men just released from Japanese prisoner-of-war camps. He was detailed to the sick bay to give assistance to the more emotionally damaged. Among the expected symptoms of grief, depression and more severe mental traumas he also found some curious reactions, one of which was that these men constantly complained about conditions on board the ship. It appeared to him that having suffered so much deprivation this complaining seemed to be part of their adjustment. But also, he thought, 'They rightly expected to receive some sympathy and understanding from their fellow servicemen, having been released from the terrible suffering they had endured. But having endured so much themselves, the other servicemen on board did not show the understanding that was expected.'

Tom Noakes applied to spend his term of national service from 1949 to 1951 in the navy. This request was disregarded and a letter informed him that he would be joining the Royal Army Medical Corps (RAMC)! At that time the length of national service was eighteen months, but during the period Tom was serving it was increased to two years, 'I was not unhappy about this as I was working in the head injury unit at Wheatley Hospital in Oxford with Sir Hugh Cairns. I then had the opportunity to work for eighteen months in the operating theatre.' During this time Tom did the entire syllabus equivalent to SRN but this counted for nothing when he returned to civilian life. There was still strong resistance to men in nursing.

Unlike Tom, Roy Stallard's first choice was the RAMC when he was called up for his national service at the age of eighteen. Earlier he had had experience as a patient on a medical ward when he suffered from paratyphoid fever. Here he had been barrier nursed in a side ward, and then placed in the open ward. Observing at first hand the day-to-day activities on the ward he had developed a keen interest in nursing. His initial RAMC training was at Queen Elizabeth's Barracks, Crookham. Here he learned the arts of marching, saluting and army discipline as well as first aid, the care of field casualties and stretcher-bearing. He was posted to British Military Hospital Munster, Germany, where he spent his two years in a typical large military hospital, in which QARANC provided the ward sisters, sister tutor and matron. The RAMC provision was for administration and the ancillary roles of quartermastering, dentistry, pharmacy and physiotherapy.

They [military hospitals] were excellent institutions, with excellent military sisters. On the wards we were always respected as members of the nursing team. The discipline was fair and no more severe than that of any ward sister I was to meet later. The training they provided me was a substantive learning curve, and as a direct result of this experience many men decided on release to further their careers in the newly formed NHS.

15 Sisters in Trousers

I was teased by my Black Country macho mates about being in a
'feminine' job, but I do not think it worried me as I could see a
future in the job.

Jeff Wood, Queen Elizabeth Hospital,
Birmingham, 1952

Up to recent years, there had always been great prejudice against men
in nursing. The lady superintendents and matrons thought male
nurses would be a threat to the moral welfare of the women, and the
hospital authorities would not allow them in their training schools.
Strong objections also came from doctors, who thought male nurses
would be a threat to their autonomy. Of the 5,700 men employed in
nursing at the beginning of the twentieth century 3,900 were working in mental hospitals. Most of the others were also looking after
mental patients, but as private nurses in the patients' own homes.
This created a unique position, with men struggling to find a role in
a female world, a role they would not establish until well after the
Second World War.

Because of these attitudes there was an almost total lack of training opportunities for men in general nursing. Although the Seamen's
Hospital, Greenwich, regularly employed male nurses on its staff, it
did not train them. The few trained nurses who were available had
picked up their limited knowledge in the asylums and infirmaries as
best they could. Other male nurses were mainly employed in private
nursing and supplied by Mr Wilson's Institute at the London
Association for Nurses, the Male Nurses' Mutual Benefit Association
or the Hamilton Association. Even with these organizations it was not
easy for men to break into nursing. There were endless rules govern-

ing their employment which did not apply to female nurses. Where employers would take female nurses completely on trust, the regulations for men were almost entirely prohibitive.

So for men the main route into nursing in civilian hospitals at the end of the nineteenth century was through asylum nursing, a discipline that was undergoing major developments. In France, Philippe Pinel was the first to set the insane free from their chains. In England, Samuel Tuke began to describe a more moral model of care at the Retreat in York. The Lunacy Act 1890 ensured that the only people to be admitted to mental hospitals were those to be certified as of unsound mind. Treatment as such was not mentioned, as there was little available. Douching with cold water, seclusion and the use of the spinning chair, where a patient was strapped in this chair and literally spun round until their behaviour was more controlled, were common. The asylum system was almost entirely custodial. The patients admitted to these hospitals suffered mainly from schizophrenia, severe depression (melancholia), mania and syphilis (general paralysis of the insane). Apart from these major mental illnesses there were admissions for some very interesting conditions: jealousy, overwork, anxiety, religious mania, disappointment in love and moral corruption (unmarried mothers).

Isolated from the community and from other disciplines asylum nursing was for many years seen as second rate. It was the growing recognition that many of their patients were curable that altered these attitudes. A more positive approach to treatment was adopted, which changed the whole approach to this speciality. But it was many years before the major breakthrough in the treatment of the mentally ill came with the introduction of tranquillizers and anti-depressants in the 1950s.

The first attempt to provide training in psychiatric nursing was in 1885 with the publication of the *Handbook for the Attendants on the Insane*. Published by the Royal Medico-Psychological Association, it was later known as the *Handbook for Mental Nurses*. It was always referred to as the Red Handbook because of the colour of the cover, and was revised and used up to the 1970s.

For a man to be successful in applying to an asylum for training for the Royal Medico-Psychological Association (RMPA) he would usually be required to be proficient at either a musical instrument or a sport; for many decades these were important attributes for anyone considering a career in this field of nursing. The entertainment and occupation of the patients were the foremost considerations, and a good staff cricket team would be highly prized by a chief male nurse. Many hospitals had their own orchestras which would play weekly for the patients and staff and monthly for the patients' ball. The requirements for admission to the RMPA was a three-year training programme with written examinations at the end of each year.

With successive mental health acts conditions gradually improved between the two world wars. The overcrowding of wards, when patients were sent to bed because there was not enough space for them in the day areas, began to be addressed. This improvement continued after the Second World War, and where there had been as many as fifty to eighty patients on a ward before the 1960s these same wards subsequently held from twenty to twenty-five patients.

A practice that was also discontinued was the ritual counting of the cutlery after the evening meal, after which the patients would line up behind their place at the table and remove their socks and shoes. Then they would remove the rest of their clothing, place them in bundles on the table, put a nightshirt on, and proceed to the dormitories and bed.

The inmates were kept occupied on the farms and in the gardens belonging to the hospital; occupational therapists began to be trained in the early 1960s. Walled airing courts were still in place in the 1960s, with nurses patrolling inside the walls to ensure that patients did not escape. Eddie Dolling remembers well the lack of structured therapy.

There was no occupational therapy available to patients until the early sixties. Up to then it was work on the farm, in the wards or in the gardens. The rest of the patients spent their time in the airing courts. On the wards the younger patients looked after the older patients and the more able older patients looked after the sick. As a charge nurse our most trusted patients almost ran the ward and kept control.

The more trusted patients would do a variety of jobs for the nurses, from car cleaning to gardening. Sister Joyce Reynolds had a patient on her ward, Madeline, who would clean and generally look after her room in the sisters' home in the grounds of the hospital. One day Joyce went to her room to get ready to go out for the night, but she could not find her corsets. She returned to the ward and asked Madeline if she had seen her corsets anywhere.'Yes sister,' she said, 'they were dirty so I washed them.' Of course they were ruined.

The main treatment for disturbed and depressed patients was therapeutic shock. Before the Second World War this was induced by insulin but In 1937 electricity began to be used; a reduced current was passed through two electrodes placed either side of the patient's forehead. Anaesthetic was not used to begin with, so the patient was awake when the electrodes and shock were applied. The intensity of the shock caused extreme rigidity of the body and could cause fractures and dislocations. Later patients were anaesthetized during this procedure. David Beech remembers the extensive use of insulin coma and abreaction with drugs such as LSD when he was on post-registration training at the Retreat in York. The introduction of chlorpromazine in 1954 quickly followed by other psychotropic drugs allowed radical changes in treatment in a wide range of mental illnesses.

Up to the 1960s there was strict segregation of the female and male sections of mental hospitals; the female side of the hospital had a matron at the head. It was recognized that the female section was run more like a general hospital. Nurses wore their distinctive uniform and were known formally as sister or nurse. On the wards, cleanliness and tidiness were as highly prized as on any general hospital ward. The sister would ensure that all able patients, nurses and orderlies were equally involved; there were no idlers. Kate Fisher well remembers her first day as a probationer nurse at the South Yorkshire Asylum in 1932, when she was presented with a set of steps and told to wash the walls as high as she could reach. The ward sister would also allocate a nurse to dormitory duties. Here there could be over eighty beds in long dormitories, with hardly any space between them. The floorboards stretched the length of the dormitory and the beds had to be lined up to those floorboards, with the wheels turned inwards. They had to have a 9-inch turnover of the sheet and perfect boxed corners; if they were not exactly right the nurse would be told to strip the lot and start again.

There were few other similarities to general hospitals, however. Kate describes her early nursing days thus: 'Every door was locked. The entire set of cutlery was counted. You stood when sister entered the ward; it was extremely strict.' As a probationer she had to live in.

Living in meant living in the side wards off the main corridor, nothing as grand as a nurses' home for us. Mainly I think it was for the benefit of the night sisters, who would call us out if a patient was being difficult. Often between the hours of seven in the morning and seven at night I would find myself delegated by sister to stand by two doors the whole shift. They were the padded cells. We were sometimes knocked about by the patients, and it could be terrifying, but that was why we had to have experienced sisters; it was from them that we gained our confidence. Mind you, I have seen many go a bit too far.

It was sister who would administer the few drugs, often with us nurses hanging on to the patient's limbs. She would kneel behind the patient, pull their head on to her lap, place a thumb at the side of the patient's mouth, force it open and pour in the medicine; the other nurse would be stroking the patient's throat to help them swallow. It sounds so crude now but the people we were dealing with were very difficult.

Kate was seventeen and a half and was paid 19s (95p) a week, with laundry and board deducted.

On the male side the hospital atmosphere was more relaxed. Surnames and very often Christian names were used – after all the charge nurse and members of his staff could be in the same cricket or football team. Male nurses originally wore caps, blue suits and waistcoats. In the 1950s they began to be issued with grey lounge suits with a waistcoat optional. These suits were well cut and were on many occasions worn outside the hospital; they graced many a wedding or funeral.

Although the male side was more informal for the staff, it was not always so for the patients. It could be almost like a barrack room, with a regimented approach to seating arrangements and mealtimes. This was not surprising, as the majority of men had come into nursing directly from the services. With no carpets, it was necessary to

202

wash and polish the floor. Chairs were usually kept in straight lines against the walls, so the tables would be moved and cleaning would commence. After washing the floor it would be bumpered. A bumper was a very heavy instrument on the end of a long pole, with a duster attached. Wax would be applied to the floor and the bumper would be swung backwards and forwards with great vigour. This was particularly useful in harnessing some of the energy of the more aggressive patients.

The dormitories were particularly regimented. Eddie Dolling remembers:

Brass taps gleamed. When chamber pots were used they were lined up handles pointed inwards under each bed. As late as the 1980s some charge nurses would still sight down the ward to ensure the beds were lined up and corners done correctly. It was not unusual to see a charge nurse crouch down to ensure correct lining of the beds.

The charge nurse needed to be resourceful when it came to maintaining harmony on the ward. This could often be achieved through the bargaining power of tobacco. The 'bacca tin' lived in the charge nurse's pocket and tobacco was doled out at his discretion. It was a control measure and a bargaining tool. On the one hand it could ensure some degree of fairness to the patients, and on the other hand tobacco could be withheld to keep them in order. There was little or no smoking on the female wards so this negotiation was achieved with snuff, which kept things ticking. For a pinch of snuff, the sister could get the heaviest and dirtiest jobs done and it was seen as a fair trade.

Meals were taken on long trestle tables, with enamel plates and mugs and so-called 'lunatic' cutlery. These were short-bladed knives and forks designed to reduce injury. Before each meal grace was said. A milestone of acceptance for a new nurse was when the charge nurse asked them to say grace. After each meal the sister or charge nurse presided over the counting of the cutlery, a custom that continued well into the 1960s. For many of the infirm elderly patients there was the dreadful 'pobs', a mixture of buttered bread, milk, and sometimes an egg mixed together in a basin. The junior nurse would go round feeding this to the helpless patients. For the sister or charge nurse, keeping the peace was a major preoccupation. With the possibility of violence ever present, a good charge nurse needed to have eyes in the back of his head, and nothing beat experience.

Under instruction from medical staff, nurses would have reasonably unfettered access to use of padded cells and straitjackets, but this became more restricted and they were eventually eliminated from mental hospitals by the end of the 1950s. All nurses carried pass keys and a whistle attached to a chain, which they lost at their peril; it was a dismissal offence.

Emergency calls were always attended to immediately. Richard Drake was new to mental nursing in the 1950s, when one day the inter-ward alarm bell rang.

The charge nurse immediately designated two other staff members and me to help out at the incident in the next ward. I ran with them, to be confronted by a patient wielding a chair above his head. He had already hit one member of staff and was certainly going to hit more, but the sheer numbers – there must have been ten of us by then – made him hesitate and with that he was restrained and removed from the area. It was all very professional and very efficient, but it took my adrenalin ages to settle.

For Eddie Dolling things got a little out of hand,

I was a student nurse. Out of the blue a patient who I thought I was developing a good relationship with attacked me. The chap punched me and pushed me up against the wall choking me; I could do nothing. Within seconds there seemed to be staff coming from everywhere. They released me and the man was removed to a side room. It was my second week in the hospital. The charge nurse tapped me on the head and said, 'Next time duck!' That was it!

Eddie Dolling also recalls, 'It was not unusual for a charge nurse to test a "doubtful" new nurse by sending them into a side room with a difficult patient to see how he coped. But there was always an experienced nurse on hand if things got a little difficult. He soon learned to look confident even if he did not feel it.' Of course incidents of this nature abound in mental nursing, but since the 1950s non-confrontational techniques of dealing with such incidents have been developed, along with improved nursing skills and the discreet use of medica tion.

From the days of the asylums, therefore, psychiatry has given men the opportunity to show their value in nursing. General nurse training on the other hand was rarely available for men before the Second World War. Only seven hospitals accepted male nurses before the war, but by the end there were twenty-four that did. This was a purely pragmatic decision, as nursing numbers were low and many men returning to civilian life wanted to continue the nursing they had learned during their service. The Society of Registered Male Nurses, formed in 1927, fought long and hard for them to be given equal status to their female counterparts. Male and female nurses did the same training but took different examinations. Where women took obstetrics and gynaecology examinations, the men took a genito-urinary (including venereal disease) examination. This effectively excluded male nurses from winning any hospital gold medals. Jeff Wood was one of the few exceptions at Queen Elizabeth Hospital, Birmingham. The Royal College of Nurses also refused to accept male nurses but by the time the Society of Registered Male Nurses was disbanded after forty years, this had changed.

The problem men had in trying to establish a role in general nursing should not be underestimated. There was almost total resistance, with many matrons vehemently opposing such an idea. At the end of the Second World War many men who had served in the medical branches of the armed services sought to further their experience in the hospitals of the day. Reg Commander answered an advertisement in the local Wolverhampton press, requesting ex-servicemen from the medical branch to apply for work on the wards at the Royal Hospital. The house governor wanted to form teams of orderlies to alleviate the nursing shortages. Having served five and a half years in the Royal Navy as a sick-berth attendant, two years as a petty officer, he felt amply suited for the job. He was in the first team and was allocated to an acute male surgical ward, being paid £5 per week. Not long after they were appointed there was a management committee meeting at which the matron proposed that they should be dispensed with. 'I do not think she liked the idea of us rough servicemen working alongside her "ladies"!' The matron was asked to reconsider her decision and her position as matron. She maintained her opinion that men should not work alongside female nurses and resigned.

The new matron seemed well disposed towards male nurses, so Reg and a colleague, Don Bentley, had their service training assessed by the General Nursing Council for state registration. The council agreed that they had met the requirements, but said they would nevertheless have to sit the preliminary and state final examinations. They approached the sister tutor, who was as intransigent as the matron who had resigned; she refused to let them use the training school, replying 'No! It isn't possible – there are girls in there!' Fortunately a more agreeable sister tutor replaced her, and they were both registered in February 1948 shortly before the introduction of the new National Health Service. To celebrate this, the house governor took Reg and Don and the two new sister tutors to dinner at the Star and Garters in Wolverhampton, followed by a box at the Hippodrome Theatre. 'They don't do things like that now, do they?' Reg mused.

Eventually Reg talked to the matron about promotion and she said she would certainly consider him. A post became available but before he applied he was sent for by the matron. She had discovered that the post was equivalent to that of sister. She told him, 'I am sorry Mr Commander but I am unable to offer you anything equal to a sister.' That evening he saw an advertisement for a charge nurse at Ivy Hospital, Cannock, and was duly promoted there.

Reg was later ordained to the non-stipendiary priesthood in 1959 and licensed to the New Cross and Wolverhampton team ministry. Some ten years ago one of the consultants at the Royal Hospital died. The new vicar asked Reg to share the service with him, and many of the consultants at the hospital attended. The vicar asked Reg if he would do the blessing at the end, and just as he was about to do so, he thought, 'I must be the only former ward orderly to have had a group of consultants on their knees in front of him.'

Tom Noakes also commenced his training at the Royal Hospital, Wolverhampton, and like Reg Commander found that misgivings about male nurses had continued into the1950s. Having been a popular student with the ward sisters he successfully passed his hospital final in 1954 and went to see the matron to receive his results. When he entered the office, the matron said, 'I see you have come first! But before we go any further you are not going to get the gold medal because it can only be given to a female nurse.' He knew this was not true, but who was he to argue with the matron?

The hospital continued to train male nurses, but when David Beech had his interview in 1956 the matron made it clear that he was welcome to train there but he should not expect a job there at the end. Coming straight from university, where he had obtained a degree in French, David was well received in the hospital, particularly as there was only one male staff nurse and one male charge nurse. This charge nurse was on permanent relief and never did have a ward or department of his own.

Like all his nursing colleagues David found the pay abysmal. In his first year he earned £210, plus meals on duty. This rose to £225 in the second year and £240 in the third year. There was a bonus of £5 for passing both parts of the examinations. During this training David recalls, 'I had the temerity to court one of the ex-staff nurses, Brenda Crane. Matron soon got to know. I not only had to seek her permission to marry but it was expected that we invite her to the wedding. She was never known to attend but there was always the dread of it!' Ten years later as a charge nurse on night duty he earned £800 per year. David had developed a keen interest in teaching and had been encouraged in this direction. Unfortunately to train as a tutor would have meant living away from home for two years. This was not practicable and so like many male nurses at that time he left nursing to take up a post as a mental welfare officer and for the first time in his life earned over £1000 per year.

During Tom Noakes's training there was one particular patient who had an influence on his future career. He was admitted with urinary problems and X-rayed, and was found to have a stone in his bladder approximately 3 inches long and 1 inch thick. It was removed and found to be a lump of calcified electric cable. The patient, who had learning difficulties, had inserted almost a yard of it into his bladder, 'I was fascinated by this and another incident and so decided that I would learn more about these people.' On completion of his state registration he commenced training in mental subnormality, as it was called then, at St Margaret's Hospital in Great Bar, Birmingham. A lot of children were admitted and he grew to like this type of work. He gained his Registered Sick Children's Nurse qualification at Great Ormond Street Hospital, London, which had just started taking men in 1955 when he started. He eventually retired at the Royal London Hospital as Senior Nursing Officer.

Following his training at Wolverhampton Royal Hospital Roy Stallard commenced an ophthalmic nursing diploma at the Eye and Ear Hospital, also in Wolverhampton, where he found a completely different attitude to promoting male nurses. Matron Jones (who died at her desk in 1975 after forty years at the hospital) wanted to encourage male nurses to become charge nurses. After only a few months as a staff nurse there he was promoted to charge nurse. Other senior posts held by male nurses at this hospital were night superintendent, theatre superintendent, male surgery, accident and emergency and out-patient department. As Roy pointed out, this was a significant male presence for 1960.

A lifetime's interest in nursing began for Tony Carr when he joined the St John Ambulance Brigade as a boy. By sixteen he had become a committed Christian and at eighteen made a decision to become a conscientious objector, leaving his occupation as a trainee engineer as it entailed working with munitions. One job that was open to him was that of a ward orderly at Selly Oak Hospital, Birmingham, and within a month he realized that his future was to be in nursing. 'One day,' he recalls, 'I was changing to go home and I suddenly had this realization that I would like to run a hospital.' But in 1950 there were no male nurses at the hospital and he did not even know that men could train as nurses. But he mentioned his ambition to a ward sister and she suggested that he should apply to the matron. He did and was accepted for training for state registration in 1951. Shortly after qualifying in 1954, two posts became available, one for a theatre staff nurse and one for a junior night sister. He went to see the deputy matron and said that he was interested in one of the posts. She asked him if he had theatre experience. He said, 'Yes, but I am interested in the night sister post.' She replied, 'Boy, you know nowt yet, you've not even grown a moustache, and you want to be night sister?' She told him to see her again in two weeks. He did, and she took him to matron. Since there had never been male nurses at the hospital before, let alone a male charge nurse, he felt his chances were bleak.

At his interview the matron said, 'You have only just qualified, Mr Carr, and I want to know if you can stand the inevitable animosity. I will do a deal with you. If you go on night duty as a staff nurse for three months and all is well, I will backdate your promotion to your first night.' It was not easy; the sister of the children's ward refused to hand the ward over to his care at night. She threatened to stay all night and the matron had to intervene on his behalf. On his first week the other night sisters completely ignored him, but slowly he was able to win them over. A year later he was promoted to senior night charge nurse.

Tony met his future wife Alice when they worked together at Selly Oak Hospital. For a married man the salary of £410 a year was insufficient for them to consider having a family. So he left and worked as a senior representative for an engineering company but could not settle to it. 'After three years I realized my first love was nursing. I wanted to return, but the only job available was trainee district nurse in Birmingham at £7 per week, and I had to provide my own car. They did provide a house for 18s 6d per week.' On completion of training he became one of the first nurses to take the new National District Nursing Certificate in 1960, having certificate No. 4. Much later he was the first male nurse to be elected to the council of the Royal College of Nursing and was appointed Principal of the William Rathbone Residential Staff College, which was opened in 1960. He retired in 1984 as Chief Nursing Officer of the Newcastle Health Authority. In 1995 he was ordained and is currently an accredited minister at the Free Methodist Church, Birmingham.

There was an increased acceptance of male nurses in general hospitals through an interchange between psychiatric nursing and general nursing from the 1950s. Many men like Eddie Dolling followed their psychiatric training with a secondment to a general hospital for state registration. Thinking that these joint skills would assist him in gaining a charge nurse post on his return to psychiatric nursing he was surprised to receive a letter from the matron offering him an immediate promotion to charge nurse of anaesthetics in the operating theatre. In the letter the matron wrote she referred to him as 'one of my boys'. Nevertheless he chose to remain in psychiatry.

Clarence Bajnath also preferred this field.

During my general nurse training, I met many nurses from the psychiatric field of nursing. With their stories and explanations about treating the whole person rather than the appendix in bed 3, or the cardiac in bed 5 I thought it would extend my own ideas about treating patients as people. I enjoyed psychiatric work although it did not always live up to my expectations about treating patients as people, particularly in terms of the elderly and long-stay patients. But custodial care was changing to a more open approach and although I was tempted to return to general nursing fortunately the 1970s was a time of great change in this area of nursing and I was pleased to stay and be part of it.

Men undoubtedly had a great deal to offer in all areas. There was an increase in the number of inter-staff marriages, but they also helped relax some autocratic attitudes and break old taboos. On the ward where Sylvia Dean worked, the sister kept all the ward stock in a locked cupboard and did not leave enough sugar, tea and biscuits out for the night. 'I was on duty and one of the male nurses picked up this problem. He took the cupboard off the wall, unscrewed the back, gave us extra rations screwed it back and hung it back on the wall. Sister may have been a little puzzled but I am quite sure she never knew what had happened.'

16   Sisters on Bicycles

To promote, through education and research, a high standard of nursing and preventative care to ensure the well-being of the nation's health; gathering and disseminating information relating to community care.

The Royal Charter laid on the Queen's Institute, 1889

The story of district nursing is over 100 years old. William Rathbone, a Liverpool philanthropist, with the support of Florence Nightingale, started this branch of nursing in 1861. Their action added a degree of legitimacy to the valuable work already being done by nurses working in the homes of the sick poor. Rathbone was so impressed by the care given to his wife by Mary Robinson, an experienced pre-Nightingale nurse from St Thomas's Hospital, that following his wife's death he encouraged Mary to nurse other people in their own homes. The people of Liverpool readily accepted the option of home care; it kept them from going into hospital. So he built and equipped a school at the Liverpool Royal Infirmary with Miss Merryweather, a graduate of the Nightingale School, as the first nurse superintendent. This school produced ward sisters, bible sisters, district nurses and private nurses. Of the first eight nurses appointed in the new branch each took one of eight districts in the Liverpool area hence the name district nurse. Only ladies were permitted to become district nurses, and their teaching was spread between district and hospital, with special instruction in home nursing. By 1874 Rathbone had founded the National Association for Trained Nurses for the Sick Poor.

In London, Florence Lees, a notable graduate of the Nightingale School, formed the East London Nursing Society in 1868, which was entered on the Rolls of Associations affiliated to the Queen Victoria

Jubilee Institute for Nurses in 1891. She was determined that the poor in this area of London should be nursed by trained and supervised district nurses. Situated on the Thames, for centuries foreigners had settled there. French, Irish and Jewish people lived side by side. This cultural mix led to some interesting cases for district nurses, not least because of the home-made treatments. One patient had a poisoned finger that had been dressed with a raw herring, another had two bad scalds, one on a hand and the other on a foot and ankle, and both were dressed with ordinary black ink! Such wounds could be highly inflamed by the time they were seen by a district nurse.

In 1887 the Queen's Nursing Institute (of district nurses) was founded, and in 1889, the year of Queen Victoria's diamond jubilee, the Institute for Nurses received its Royal Charter. Rosalind Paget, a niece of William Rathbone, was Number 1 on the Queen's Roll of Nurses. She was later made a dame and appointed Inspector General of the Institute.

Florence Nightingale was well aware of the difference between nursing in a hospital, with its supportive systems of discipline and control, and working in the community on one's own in someone else's home. She wrote in her notes of 1876, *Trained Nurses of the Sick*, that the district nurse should be of a higher class than a hospital nurse and more fully trained. She argued that the community doctor had to rely on her fully to act as his clinical clerk by reporting the condition of the patient, as a wound dresser, and as a nurse. She further explained that besides nursing the patient, the district nurse should also show them how they could call in official sanitary help to make the 'poor room' healthy, how they could improvise appliances, and how the home need not be broken up because of poverty. She must be a nurse, suggested Miss Nightingale, but she must also nurse the room, in cleanliness, in ventilation, and in removing any sorts of foulness.

Preparing the sick room was most important, as many operations were performed in the patient's home. Dr Humphrey wrote in *A Manual of Nursing* in 1891 that slight operations could be performed in the patient's own bed having ensured that it had been previously arranged and with a rubber mackintosh sheet to protect the floor from the blood. For greater operations, or those which took longer or required good light, an operating table could be devised. A firm wooden table such as a dressing table or kitchen table was thought to answer the purpose, provided it was strong and steady. This, he suggested, should be furnished with blankets, pillows and mackintosh sheets, arranged in the following way. The table was best placed in a room with a good light, and near the window. It was thought convenient to use a room adjoining the bedroom so that the patient could not see the preparation of the instruments, but could receive the anaesthetic in bed, and then be carried into the 'operating room'. A fire was to be prepared to provide constant hot water and warmth to avoid shock.

Miss Nightingale wanted the district nurse to be a caseworker and a supervisor of the poor rather than a provider for them. She was not there to act for the patients but to direct help to support them. In this, district nursing initially had an uncomfortable relationship with the medical profession. The suspicion was that these well-educated, knowledgeable and professional ladies could usurp the doctors in the houses of the poor and thus deprive them of part of their income. This was not the case, however, and steadily a unique partnership grew between nursing and medicine.

Reports abound of unconditional caring by district nurses. In 1901, the mother of a girl with a hip disease died, leaving her child without care. No hospital was able to help so a district nurse was sent. She provided nursing care and assistance for the girl in the house, and later arranged for her to attend a 'cripple school' daily. Another young woman of twenty-four contracted typhoid fever, complicated by pneumonia, and became delirious. The doctor considered her situation was too serious to move her to hospital and sent for a district nurse to attend her. For eighteen days she nursed her at home until she could be admitted to hospital, where she stayed for two months. On discharge the nurse again attended her for thrombosis, possibly caused by prolonged bed rest. An 'assistant lady' provided coal for the fire and help in providing blankets, extra food, and medical supplies – the district nurse was expressly instructed never to provide anything of this kind herself. There were also many children with infectious diseases complicated by pneumonia who were unable to gain hospital admission and needed the skilled care of the district nurse. The compassion of nursing is clearly evident in these cases, with the district nurse providing as much social support as nursing.

Alice Ashworth took the Queen's Institute of District Nursing examination on 20 September 1934. These four questions from the paper show the issues that were relevant then.

1. What is the difference between a deep and a shallow well? What difference might you expect to find in the water obtained from them and why? What precautions would you advise to be taken in time of drought when water has to be obtained from unreliable sources?
2. What preparations would you make for an operation on a child for the removal of tonsils in a patient's home? What after-care would you expect to give as a district nurse and what advice should be given?
3. How can the organism of tuberculosis gain admission to the human body and in what parts of the body does the disease usually appear in infants, children and adults?
4. What facilities are available for dealing with?
    (a) underfed school children;
    (b) an old age pensioner needing medical attention;
    (c) a factory girl needing a change of air after a severe illness;
    (d) a child obviously suffering from neglect?

The first district nurses, with their unmistakable special cloaks and bonnets were usually provided with a bicycle and later a motorcycle to assist them in their work. As honoured contributors to the health and well-being of local people, it was safe for district nurses and midwives to travel alone throughout the country, apart from in wartime. The problem then was that shattered glass constantly punctured their bicycle tyres. In the East End of London one man devoted his time to repairing the nurses' tyres as his contribution to the war effort.

The nurses needed their mobility. Miss Clunn was a district nurse midwife who was regularly called to help mothers giving birth, irrespective of the bombing going on around them. One night she was called to a confinement in a block of flats in Hackney, where there was heavy damage all around. In the flat there were no windows, no lighting, no heating, and no water. By the light of a carefully veiled torch, twin babies were delivered as the bombs fell. Within a short time she was on the top floor of Beecham Tower in the Tower of London. The mother was already in labour when falling bombs made it too dangerous to stay there, so she was moved to the ground-floor kitchen. The mother and baby both survived, as did Miss Clunn.

Joan Jenkins commenced her nurse training on 1 January 1934 at St George's Hospital, London, the same day as Muriel Powell. By the 1950s she had made a decision to work as a district nurse and went to Sheffield. There was a new estate being built and she was offered a house, where she still lives. She was only there a matter of hours when a young boy came to the door and said, 'Can you come quick, me mum says me granny's conked out.' It was the start of many wonderful years on this district, where she could leave her bicycle anywhere and never needed to lock her door. She said, 'I used to keep bedpans, urinals, and other equipment in my outhouse and anyone could come and borrow what they wanted. I knew it would all be returned.' She always laid out the bodies of her patients at death. 'They were still my patients you see!' She explained, 'I set out every morning and went to the very ill first, you bathed them and made them comfortable. Then there would be injections, dressings, and people coming out of hospital sometimes with terrible wounds, but we did not have infection in the district once we had cleaned these wounds up.'

At the age of sixty-four when the authorities realized that she was four years over pensionable age she was asked to retire. The doctor she had worked with at the local surgery told her that they had a position for someone to do dressings and help at reception if she would like to continue working. 'I did. I did three days a week, then reduced to two. When I was eighty-three I said to them, "I think I had better leave as I can't read very well now." The other staff said, "Well come and make the coffee we will cover for you." I did this for another two years.'

In her district in Lancashire, Alice Ashworth went to an eighteen-year-old who was confined to her bed. She lived with her father, who was at work all day.

My first job was to put the kettle on and light a fire. I would get her washed and get her something to eat. I had another girl with the same condition, who was in constant pain when

215

moved; both these patients had rheumatic fever, very common in the 1930s and 1940s. I had to do everything for them. My experience as a fever nurse nursing diphtheria cases who also could have heart complications stood me in good stead. In the isolation wards of the fever hospital we would nurse these people so that they did not have to do anything that would cause strain on the heart.

Alice was also called to a home to attend a mother in labour late one night, the labour was progressing slowly; and, as the mother had had normal births previously, she was quite concerned. The GP decided to apply forceps so Alice was given a metal face-mask and gauze for the patient and told to drip chloroform over it. As the mother was sedated and began to relax the baby emerged unaided but sadly was diagnosed as anencephalic (neural tube defect) and died. These days such abnormalities are simply prevented by taking folic acid.

Lucy Baird (née Simon) explained that one of the villages she went to in her 20-mile circuit as a district nurse was up a long steep hill. At the top was a sort of post box where people from the village left letters informing her if they needed a visit. If they could not get to the post box someone would do it for them. 'Well this was fine for a while until one day I opened the box and out popped a mouse. I am terrified of mice and when I saw the superintendent I said no more, I am not going all that way to have mice jumping out at me, they will have to get a telephone fixed, and they did.'

Her district had other hazards. She was called to one house where the mother lived upstairs and the rest of the family downstairs; they had two large dogs. She had been upstairs to see to the mother and came down to prepare a dressing for her ulcerated leg. Her dog, a much-loved German shepherd, was very put out that Lucy had been in the bedroom alone with its owner while it had been ushered away. She started to prepare the dressing in the kitchen.

In the 1940s, we used an American preparation, antiflijustin, which later changed to kaolin for poultice dressings. I was pasting this on, and the dog suddenly launched himself at my neck. Luckily the family pulled it off but I still needed seven sutures.

216

I was given two aspirin and allowed two days off.

On another of her visits she received a gift of one of the first fold-up umbrellas.

When I arrived the family were all standing round a large fluffy cat. 'We've got a favour to ask,' they said. 'We've done mother just as you told us to but the cat has got all messed up, she's been out all night. We wondered if you would please wash her.' So I duly dunked Snowball in the sink with she protesting vigorously and then I went to see how my patient was. You did things like that in those days, nobody would object and that was how I got my very first fold-up umbrella.

When visiting patients at home, district nurses were advised to put their coats on a newspaper to prevent carrying infection around with them. Alice Ashworth explained.

On entering the patient's house, we were told never to put our nursing bag on the floor, always on a table. To take off our coat and fold it inside out, and never hang it behind a door or in the hall adjacent to other clothing, and we were never to sit on a chair which was upholstered or on which there was a cushion. These instructions were given to avoid the transference of vermin from one patient's house to another, and of course to us. We were also instructed to respect the patient's possessions, for example, never put a bowl of very hot water on an unprotected polished surface such as a table or chest.

Many nurses concluded that three months on the district could give them more insight into how their patients lived than three or four years in a hospital. Poverty was rife, both in the country and in the inner cities. Here a nurse learned about how people lived as well as how they dealt with their sickness and cared for their sick at home. Lucy Baird went to a house and found the family having an argument. The patient was upstairs, very ill, and when she got to him she found the sheet he was lying on was wet through. She did not want to go down again and face the argument.

I looked around for some sheets, but there were none. On the dressing table was a white cloth with a statue on. I moved the statue (the Madonna) aside and used the cloth as a sheet. When I had finished I went down and told the family what I had done. There was an immediate silence then an outcry of, 'Oh my, that is the holy cloth.' They were more concerned about the cloth than the poor man upstairs.

On another occasion one of the nurses she worked with had prepared for a visit from her supervisor, only to be told at the last minute that it had been cancelled. Although she was relieved, it was very unusual for a visit to be cancelled, so she asked why. She was informed that all three supervisors were ill with stomach pains. It appears that one of them was taking her turn to cook. She made up a stew, and in it she sliced what she thought was an onion – it seems that she could not tell the difference between onion and daffodil bulbs.

Patients had to pay for visits from the district nurse, and there were various clubs to which they could pay a few pennies a week; they would then get a district nurse or hospital care if they were ill. One of the first questions the nurse asked was whether the patient had paid into the club or not. In Bolton and many cities it was called the Saturday Fund and some still exist today, albeit in a different form since 1948. As the service ran on subscriptions and voluntary donations, district nurses often involved themselves in fund-raising events.

The district midwife has also had a unique role in the community. 'Nursing in the district is different to nursing in hospital, and midwifery in the district is different again,' said Dorothy Turner. 'When nursing in a hospital you are awaiting instructions from a doctor but in midwifery working in the community you are on your own; you have to diagnose, deliver and prescribe.'

Up to the end of the Second World War contraception was not a subject that was openly discussed in the home or at school, nor did it rate very highly in any community discussions – certainly not in inner cities, where ignorance prevailed. So for a community midwife some situations could be very complex. In most cases when a girl became pregnant, because of social and family pressures the boy would marry her. When this did not happen the shock of having an unmarried mother in the family would be extreme – so profound, in fact, that many families kept their daughters indoors from the moment the first physical signs showed. The girls would only be allowed out at night when the 'bump' was less visible. At full term the daughter would be despatched to an aunt or grandmother for the birth. There are many examples of babies being taken over by another family member; in many cases this involved pretending that the baby was the girl's mother's. These were the lucky ones, however. In far too many cases girls would be confined to an asylum as morally corrupt. Many women spent their entire lives locked in institutions simply because of pregnancy before wedlock; the stories are many and heartbreaking. In the early twentieth century society had exacting standards of acceptable behaviour and social isolation was also the lot of mothers who had babies in later life – thirty-five onwards. These women, particularly in deeply religious communities, were ashamed to admit that at their age they were still having sex.

Bella Blandford remembers men being more involved in the birth of a baby at home than is often acknowledged. They were banned from hospital confinements, but this was not the case in the community. Apart from the inevitable boiling of water and making cups of tea, the father would almost always help. 'We delivered with the mother on her side or on her back, so if I was on my own, which I often was, someone would have to hold the mother's leg. You could have one leg over your shoulder and the other held by the father. Quite often the granny would do this if the father was not available.' Mothers to be were induced in a variety of ways. Castor oil, enemas, and hot baths were fairly normal. A tight binder was also often carefully wrapped round the bulge and held with numerous safety pins. At this time it was not unusual to burn the placenta and dressings in the garden.

After the Second World War conditions in slum areas of inner cities had changed little from the previous century. Shared outside lavatories were common, as were communal taps, and many district nurses and midwives had to rely on them for water. They would be sure of a warm welcome, however, and with large families commonplace the midwife would also be sure of regular visits. Gladys Boots, who trained at the North Middlesex Hospital, remembers:

Working as a district midwife in an inner city was challenging. I met so many poor families with very few material possessions. In those days they would rely on the parish or national assistance for support, it was a humiliating experience. None of the patients had phones, so if I needed the doctor or the 'flying squad' I had to go out and use a public phone. But I found it so rewarding delivering a baby in the family's home.

Radiotelephones were not introduced into the health service until the late 1960s. They consisted of a receiver and transmitter. Susan Eardley-Stiff, a midwife working in Portsmouth, described their introduction as 'a wonderful innovation to us'.

From a midwife's point of view they were brilliant, not only in the ease of communication but also in terms of safety for the midwife. Controlled from an ambulance station the midwife could be contacted in an emergency and she could also rapidly co-ordinate support with medical and other services from the patient's home. Patients in the more deprived area did not have telephones in their homes.

Unfortunately, in terms of safety, times were changing and leaving a notice on the midwife's door with a list of where they would be for the day was becoming less safe. When Susan was a trainee on the district in Southampton, she was on a night visit with the district nurse. The husband had called them but when they arrived he was not there. When they asked where he was the mother told them he was at work. They delivered the baby and when they returned to the midwives' home it had been burgled. When the police arrested the man involved, it was the husband of the new mother.

When Gladys Boots was district nursing in the Romford area she was somewhat shocked with one family, where the father was a coffin-maker.

When the baby was delivered I asked them for somewhere to place him. The mother said, 'Put him in there.' It was a child's coffin. I said, 'No way; he is not going in there.' I gave the baby back to the mother, took the coffin out into the hall and pulled

220

a drawer out of the dressing table. I put a blanket and sheets inside and placed the baby in it. The family could not see what the problem was.

Nor could the midwife she was standing in for. She had seen into the world a number of the family's children, and each one spent their first days of life in a coffin.

Parent-craft classes were much needed additions to social education, and Elsie Joel ran one such class on Tyneside. One of the young men who attended was very supportive to his wife and wanted to be at the unit when the baby was born. Unfortunately he worked at a pit 5 miles under the North Sea and 20 miles from the unit. The mother's time duly arrived. Having already phoned her husband, she would not co-operate until he arrived. Elsie, however, still had a baby to deliver. So it was with great relief she heard footsteps and a male voice outside the labour ward. She opened the door and a young man in jeans and jumper asked for the patient by name. 'I asked if he was the father and when he said yes, I was so relieved I took him straight into the labour ward. He did not get the reception I expected; the mother screamed instead of welcoming him in her undignified position – he was the father of their local Catholic church.'

The defining point for a pupil midwife was her first home delivery. The district sister would take out a new pupil, and when she was happy the pupil would then accompany a senior before attending her first birth on her own. Another defining point was the expectant parent's first child. This was the happy moment for John and Barbara Samuels. Thinking it would be a good idea to light a fire in the bedroom, John only managed to fill the room with smoke, as the chimney was blocked with soot. An obviously new but very pleasant pupil midwife arrived and prepared the bed, only for a rather severe sister midwife to follow, strip it, and tell the pupil to make it again and make it properly. All this time John was boiling water.

I had no idea why I was doing this, but this is what people did. I was even more surprised later when I realized that the hot water I kept taking to the bedroom door disappeared, never to be seen again. Of course I was never allowed in myself. What they did with all that water I never did find out!

Important in home delivery were the confidences shared between the mother and the midwife. It was often the only opportunity a mother had, for example, to explain that the baby was not the husband's. At one delivery a mother seemed to be in pain, and the husband was quite distressed. Susan Eardley-Stiff found it unusual for a mother in labour to scream out with pain in her own home. She sent the husband to the car to get some gas and air. The mother immediately stopped her screaming and looked almost relieved that she could relax for a moment. Susan asked her what the matter was, and the girl replied, 'This is not my first baby but I am having to make out that it is; it's harder work than actually having the baby.'

Alice Carr (née Smith) trained at Selly Oak Hospital, Birmingham, from 1950 to 1953. She soon decided that district midwifery was for her. One of her early placements was in the Erdington district with Miss Alice Briggs.

I was the last one to do my midwifery training with her and throughout that training I had to live at her house. I was courting my future husband, Tony, also a nurse. Miss Briggs would allow me to have him in the house in the evening but I had to be in my uniform because I was always on duty. He would call and Miss Briggs would invite him in and tell him where to sit and we would talk. Then at ten sharp she would say, 'It is ten o'clock and time for you to go.' Then she would turn to me. 'Now say goodnight. You can have five minutes but don't shut the door.' Then off he would go; I was twenty-four years old! We married a year later.

On one occasion when she was still under instruction, Miss Briggs told Alice to meet her at a certain house. Alice arrived first, so she went to the bedroom and there was the mother.

When I pulled the sheets back, there was an eight pound baby. What a shock; I did not know at this time that things like that could happen. It became 'my' first baby. When you delivered a baby, under instruction or not, those mothers and babies were yours. So if you delivered three that week you would have to visit each one every day for fourteen days. You would have to swab the mum, check their nipples and uterus, and bath the baby. Over a Christmas period I had twenty deliveries in twenty-two days. As you can imagine, I was working all day and at night.

Alice also pointed out that until recent years if there were no complications women almost always wanted to have their babies in their own homes. For this the midwife would have to be satisfied that they had enough clothing for the baby. In the poor area where she worked she knew there would be a bundle of clothes ready at each house, but it had been borrowed and passed around from mother to mother. This borrowing was a tradition that went back to the Victorians. In many poor areas a box or package was kept, usually in the local vicarage, with nighties, napkins, long flannel vests, tiny sewn tops, swaddling bandage and swathes. These were loaned for the first few weeks following the birth and always returned, fully laundered, to the vicarage.

On one occasion, when Miss Briggs was going on leave, she left Alice instructions about a patient that she expressly wanted visiting. It was her tenth baby. 'When I visited her I said, "You are due this week." "Oh no my dear," she said, "I am not having this baby until Miss Briggs is back." "But you are already overdue," I argued. It made no difference. "No, not until Miss Briggs is back!" So we agreed that I would visit every day. The baby was duly born on Miss Briggs's first day back from leave. As it happened there were complications that Alice knew she would have had difficulties with. 'I thought it amazing what mind over matter could do!'

Avril Vincent also lived in the district nurses' home, but with her friend Jenny. They moved to the Gosport district after training at the Royal Hampshire Hospital, staying at the house of Mrs and Miss Petigrew. Avril was assigned to Miss Petigrew. When this lady was promoted to be matron of Blake House Maternity Home in Gosport, she took both Avril and her friend with her. Miss Petigrew informed them both that she did not approve of them staying for more than a year; she thought by then they should be gaining further experience. Nineteen years later Avril finally left to gain a post as nursing officer at St Mary's Hospital maternity unit, Portsmouth.

For Gwen Savage working with the district midwife was the most enjoyable part of her training.

During my general training we were assigned to a district midwife in a very rural area and had to stay overnight in her cottage. It was a different world. She made her own decisions regarding her daily round and her visits were often the highlight of someone's day. Methods of sterilization were often primitive and one learned how to improvise.

She noticed how often the midwife would invite the husband to be present during childbirth. They had to be alert to changes in the colour of the husband's face, however, to avoid having another patient at a vital time.

Gwen soon realized that as a district nurse she would be able to make her own decisions and could change her practice without first seeking permission. So after further training she applied and was given her own district in a mining area in the Tyne valley. Moving to a house on the main road she became used to the sound of miners' clogs and sticks as they made their way to and from the pits, but it took a little longer for her to get used to the dialect and way of life. The strength of the bond between members of these tight-knit mining communities, their subculture and extended family structures made for powerful support networks. If on one of her pre- or post-natal visits the patient happened to be out, she would simply go to her mother's house; she was almost guaranteed to find her there.

In the more rural parts of her district it took considerable courage to drive across fields in the dark of winter to remote farm cottages with no electricity, then deliver a baby. It was not unusual to have a 'pit-man's ration' (a sack of coal) in the back of her car to give extra weight on the back axle when it snowed. As she said, 'They were canny folk up there!' In these outer areas her home and the local pub acted as the casualty department. Here swabs were baked in a tin in the oven, instruments were sterilized in a saucepan, and 'we did not have problems with infection'.

Attending a birth with no gas or electricity and only a fire and oil lamp was one problem, but changing outdated attitudes was quite another. One day following a normal birth, she found that the baby had been tightly swaddled and was hypothermic. These practices were common: the patient's mother, her grandmother and her great-grandmother had done this so this mother was determined to do it too. The family took some convincing that reasonable freedom of movement for the baby was essential.

Something nurses never forget is the death of a new-born baby, whether at home or in hospital. These rare occurrences were all the more tragic when the birth was uncomplicated. Dorothy Turner went to a particular lady and delivered a girl, Zoe. After three boys the mother was delighted to have a girl, and both were fine. When she called the next morning, however, the mother said that Zoe had not woken and she was a little worried.

I went to see what was wrong and could see that she was not moving. I said, 'Zoe, Zoe what is wrong?' It may seem silly to say this but you got so attached to the family. I immediately took her to the hospital, where nothing could be done; the baby died. I still think of Zoe, she would be twelve or thirteen now. I have delivered all sorts of abnormal and still births, but the hardest is a normal birth when the baby dies. I went to the funeral and that was very difficult.

Margaret Webster's main patch was Brixton and Stockwell in London, where there was a mixture of English, West Indian and Irish.

Being sister I always seemed to have pupils with me, so I decided I would do one call on my own. I went to this house and there was a West Indian lady waiting with her coat and hat on. Knowing how scrupulously clean these people were I was not at all concerned about delivering in the house, which was just as well as she was within moments of having her baby. I hustled her back into the house and into a downstairs room where there was a bed. Ignoring her protests, and with her hat still on, the baby was delivered. The bed happened to be the landlady's and when she returned she was not at all pleased with the happy event.

One night when Margaret Morris and a friend were pupil

midwives training in London, the district midwife was called out to an imminent delivery at midnight.

We were told to locate the house and not be late. Feeling quite safe even at that time of night we set out on our bikes armed with our bags. We chatted the whole way, got to the street, and neither of us could remember the number of the house. We cycled along the street and fortunately found a house with a light on in an upstairs bedroom window. Somewhat in a panic by now we decided this had to be it. We knocked and an old man answered the door; he was well in his eighties. Instantly we knew we had the wrong house and tried to explain, only to be answered with, 'Can't a man get up in the night for a pee without you waking the whole dammed street up?'

Throughout her career Elsie Joel felt comfortable travelling anywhere on her bicycle.

I was never afraid, never at risk; children would come to my door saying, 'My mum wants you now!' or in the night dads would come for me and although I had never met them before I was never at risk; they would carry the gas and air and I had the black bag. When there was fresh snow we would link arms and slip and slide around together. One came for me on his powerful motorbike and I had to ride pillion. 'Lean with the bike nurse,' he said. I was sure my weight and a bag under each arm would tip me off.

Following many of these adventures she was often offered small gifts of fresh fish or a lobster fresh from the quayside on the Tyne, usually still alive, or fresh flowers and vegetables dug from the garden. 'I would rarely come away empty-handed.'

Elsie's district was a working class area of Tyneside. Proud to be a midwife, she felt greatly respected and confident in her district nurse uniform. Every day she rode her bicycle, with the black bag on the back, across a busy main road. There was a police box on the corner, which usually had a couple of constables inside. If they saw her approaching, one of them would dash out, put his white gloves on, stop the traffic and wave her across. They would exchange greetings as she passed and off she would go, feeling quite important. She always thought this was because she was the district midwife, an important member of the community delivering babies at home, day and night. Many years later, however, that she met one of these constables, now an inspector, at a wedding. She approached him and said, 'I remember you, you always used to stop the traffic for me on Borough Street when I was on my bike.' He grinned and said he remembered her very well. 'As you know,' he said, 'there were always two of us in the box and when we saw you coming down the hill we would toss a coin to see whose turn it would be. When you cycled across that junction you pedalled so fast we could see your suspenders.'

17 Night Duty Sisters

The night nurse should be on duty twelve hours, with instant
dismissal if found asleep and four hours for daily exercise or
private occupation . . . I do not fancy, but at present am not positive about, cleaning or scrubbing at night.

Florence Nightingale, *Subsidiary Notes*

There was an old music hall joke about the night sister: 'Wasn't she
the one who woke you up at night to give you a sleeping tablet?'
Night sisters were affectionately or otherwise known as the 'queen
bee' from evening till morning. Until the nineteenth century there
were no queen bees, as there were no nurses in attendance at night.
In the eighteenth century watchers were present during the night, and
watching is what they did. They lived outside the hospitals, were not
trained, and were from the least favoured part of society. By the nineteenth century, however, night nurses began to be employed and day
nurses would work nights in rotation, with a consequent improvement in this aspect of care. The main function of these nurses was to
provide clean chamber pots for the patients, visit the most ill regularly and ensure the ill-nourished patients ate their prescribed feeds.
Later, night sisters were employed and they would do at least three
rounds a night; if they found a problem they would call out the ward
sister from her room next to the ward. On most wards there were
two large fires, one at each end; it was the night nurse's duty to keep
them lit, and many nurses were dismissed because they let the fire go
out; it was deemed that they must have been sleeping on duty.

Night duty at the time when Florence Nightingale began her
reforms was extremely arduous. The nurses' duties would begin at
7.00 a.m. They would attend to the needs of the patients during that

day until 5.00 p.m., then they could rest until 10.00 p.m. They would then be on duty all night and day until the following evening. There would be time for food breaks, but no other rest periods. After one night's sleep they would be up again and on duty at 7.00 a.m., working through until 10.00 p.m. The same cycle of duty would commence the very next morning. This may be an extreme example, but at most hospitals it was a twenty-hour period of duty with only short periods of rest. The nurse would have one week's leave per year, increasing to two after four years' continuous service. One of a night nurse's duties would be cooking the night sister's supper. Unless the nurse had already had her cookery course in the kitchen, this could well be her first venture into cooking. Scrambled eggs were one thing, cooking raw meat such as bacon, lamb's liver and kidney would be quite another. One can only guess at the burnt offerings the night sisters would have had, but they resolutely carried this tradition out for many years.

The camaraderie of night duty has always been special. It was a singularly different world from the day. There was little time for boredom; the day sister would have ensured that. Nurses inevitably had more responsibility and freedom to make their own decisions, but always with the safety net of having the night sister to call on. Emergencies during the night were inevitable with operations, collapses, haemorrhages and road accidents. Some nights the operating theatre could be in constant use, and depending on the size of the hospital the night sister could spend a considerable time there.

Hospitals were always short of staff, so it was imperative that night nurses reported for duty. Margaret Marsh was at King's College Hospital, London, in the awful smog of the 1950s and had to walk from the nurses' home in Dulwich to the hospital in Camberwell. One night it was particularly bad. The matron and a group of medical students came to the home with lamps. The nurses were organized into a crocodile procession, with one hand on the shoulder of the person in front. 'To us it was all very exciting. The medical students loved it and of course we were all very young, very giggly girls. We did not at the time realize the implications for the people living through it year after year, there were so many who suffered and died.'

Later in her career it always amazed Margaret that the job of night sister was thought to suit a new sister. She disagreed. 'When you think of the field they have to cover and the responsibility it is a horrendous job for new sisters. Being responsible for 130 patients is a huge responsibility. I liked the communication one had with the staff; they were regular staff and you got to know each one.'

As a night sister, Mary Hearn felt she had an average responsibility on night duty with seven wards to look after; three surgical, two gynaecology and two ear nose and throat. The division was geographical rather than by speciality. Her first job would be to go round and work out the night priorities, check the theatre and look at the new admissions. She talked to each patient; in this way she got to know them very well. Each night sister had her own controlled drugs in a locked box that she carried with her:

The hysterectomy patients would be on pethidine for pain relief every four hours. This meant a regular visit to the ward, which was all right until you had a really busy night with surgical emergencies and such, then it came to the morning and you found one ampoule short. You then had to go round the wards checking and rechecking. Sometimes it could be ten in the morning before I could go off duty.

They also had to make major decisions and take instruction regarding controlled drugs over the phone. 'If someone had a major crisis I would take instructions to give morphine. I had to, there was no one else there. We could act on verbal messages.'

Operating theatres still worked at night, and that was when domestic cleaning was done. The nurses' home also had to be secured and rounds had to be undertaken. There were also some unusual duties. Former workhouse infirmaries were altered at the introduction of the NHS in 1948 to accommodate elderly patients. However, many of them still had cottages in their grounds where people who had no accommodation could stay. Mothers and children went into these, and the men had to sleep separately in the tramps' section. It was the night sister's job to ensure that the men were out of the cottages before lights out. She would be expected to go round each cottage to check the rooms, including the wardrobes and under the beds to ensure that no one was trying to stay the night.

Night sisters at St Thomas's Hospital have traditionally been known as 'night asses'. This was not a surprising nickname when one considers how far one of these sisters might have to travel in a night. To measure this Daphne Fallows was fitted with a pedometer and was measured as travelling 14 miles; that same night, another sister was measured as travelling nearly 20 miles. This included climbing stairs, as the use of lifts was not allowed at night. There were three floors to cover from 9.00 p.m. to 8.00 a.m. 'Thank goodness the floors were wooden, not concrete,' she said.

One nursing absurdity has been the traditional feuding between day and night staff. Neither could quite do the job to the satisfaction of the other. This animosity could get out of hand on occasions, and it inevitably meant that the night nurses suffered. It was they who would be called back from their rooms to rectify an error or omission, no matter how trivial. Apart from the night superintendent, the night sister was usually junior to the ward sisters, and a junior night sister with a 'bolshie' reputation would have difficulty gaining promotion to a day sister post. One ward sister was a terror to the night staff, as Sheila Grant recalls. Known as the 'bantam hen' she was only 5 feet tall.

But my goodness you knew she was there. When she entered the ward in the morning she would strut around talking to all the patients, but all the time noting the beds. If there was one corner not folded correctly, she would strip the bed back with, 'Nurse, make that bed properly before you go off duty.' She would also put her hand in every bed to ensure that the patient was dry, and there would be hell to pay if she found a wet sheet.

Working night duty could be very tiring. Wendy Carson was working nights on a very busy surgical ward. One night it was so bad she barely had time to sit down at all except to write the report. But the sister expected a personal report when she arrived in the morning. For a start Wendy was in her bad books because she had kept her waiting. Wendy always dreaded the procedure.

This involved placing the report in front of her while she sat at her desk, then standing behind her and reading the report out loud over her shoulder. I nearly fell asleep on my feet looking down trying to read; then I started missing words. Each time she would stop me and make me read it again. Finally I said to her that I was just too tired and asked her if she could read it herself, so she did!

She asked a few questions as she read and then told Wendy to go and get some sleep. 'The next night was just as busy,' she remembers. 'But the following morning when I went into the office to give the report, there was a chair for me to sit alongside her, also a cup of tea. I still had to read the report which she had in front of her.'

Telephones were in commercial use from 1877 and widely introduced into hospitals in the 1880s, but at many hospitals they were not used between 8.00 p.m. and 6.00 a.m. The use of lifts during the night, apart from emergencies, was also discouraged. These two initiatives were aimed at keeping the noise down, and continued until recent years. However, anyone who has ever been in hospitals at night will know that bedpans and trolleys made up for any reduction in peripheral noises.

Activity on the wards started from as early as 4.00 a.m. From that time on there was an inevitable build up of pace. Specimen jars had to be readied, pots of tea made, bread sliced for toast, and special diets, trolleys and trays to be prepared. At 5.00 a.m. it was time for the most junior nurse to start the trip down to the kitchen to collect the porridge. In winter it was quite a trial walking along cold, dismal corridors. The nurse would then have to deliver to all the other wards in her area. At 6.00 a.m. the real day would begin. In between the four-hourly routines of back rounds, blood pressures, temperatures and dressings, there was also the bedpan round, and washing bowls and tooth mugs to be cleaned. The bed-making round completed, there was a night report to be written. At 8.00 a.m. the night nurse would report to the day sister and if anything was not done to the sister's satisfaction, then the nurse had to stay until it was. Nurses soon learned not to hand over a task they were involved in just so that they could go off duty on time; if it was started while they were on duty they finished it.

An experiment on two wards at St George's Hospital in the 1950s led to the end of early-morning waking for patients throughout the country. When Muriel Powell was matron of the hospital, she encouraged two ward sisters to alter the routines that had led to early waking. Where previously it was common practice for patients to be woken at 5.00 a.m., this was changed to 7.00 a.m., but not without a great deal of resistance. Joan Jenkins remembers:

Her argument was that the wards should be run for the convenience of the patients. Cleaning times were altered and so was the consultant's rounds. She said they should be content with many of the patients being bathed during their rounds instead of first thing in the morning. There was initial resistance but also an enthusiasm to try this very revolutionary approach to patient care.

The night sister had at her disposal one or more of the junior nurses who acted as 'runner' between wards. She did not work on any particular ward, but would be sent to any area requiring extra assistance, normally to assist in turning heavy patients, relieving breaks and filling gaps. It was not always a popular role, but it did provide variety and an opportunity to hear the current gossip or pass on any titbits the nurse had gleaned during her travels.

Some night sisters seemed to have more authority than the matron did. The nurses' home at Queen Alexandra Hospital, Cosham, where Mary Hearn trained had a special corridor for the night staff. Night nurses had to be in bed by 9 30a.m., and the night sister would be there to ensure that they were. In the summer the young nurses really wanted to be out in the sun, but they had to be in their beds. Mary said:

If you came out of your room before four in the afternoon, she was there, and back you would go. She had a list so she knew who was and was not on duty. When she got her own sleep I do not know. In the summer you could not get sunburned – it was a self-inflicted injury; if you did, on duty you would go. You soon learned not to mention it even when in agony all night.

The nurses had half an hour's break in the night and she would check that they had something to eat. 'She seemed to spend more of her time checking us nurses than the patients.' Not only that, between

10.00 p.m. at night and midnight she would position herself on the top corridor, overlooking the entrance to the hospital (which included the local cinema). Here she would sit watching the nurses returning with their boyfriends. They had to be back by 10.30 and she knew who had a late pass. These nurses also knew she would be watching so they ensured that she would not see them kissing their boyfriends goodnight. She took her role as moral guardian very seriously.

The night sister's ward-rounds were dreaded just as much as the matron's and she would expect her nurses to have some knowledge of all the patients by her 10.00 p.m. round – their name, diagnosis and treatment. Daphne Fallows acknowledged how sorry she felt for the nurses, who hardly had time to get sorted out, 'and along I would come wanting to know all this information.' During these rounds many nurses tried making things up but they rarely got away with it; sister had done her homework from the ward reports. It always amazed new nurses that the night sister could have knowledge of as many as seven or eight wards full of patients.

Woe betide the nurse who was caught with her cape over her shoulders while doing any work with patients. It meant that she had either been sitting in her chair with it round her shoulders, or that she had not removed it after her break time. If a nurse relaxed too much, a testy voice would say, 'Have you not noticed that Mr A is awake and in pain?' One night duty Derek Bates found that he had what is called 'phantom legs'. It was 3.00 a.m., the worst time for any night nurse. Seeing the night sister coming towards him he jumped from his chair only to find her suddenly towering some distance above him. He pulled himself as upright as he could but it made no difference.

Knowing I was not dreaming I tried to move and it was at this point that I realized that I was in fact 'stood' on my knees. Night Sister spun round and disappeared from the ward. She returned some ten minutes later, then had me escort her round the ward. She never once mentioned the incident.

Although one of her roles was to ensure that all the nurses were awake and alert, the night sister did not always manage this herself. Audrey Jones (later Watts) remembered: 'We called Night Sister

"Bootsy", as she always came on duty wearing black boots, she looked hilarious with her sister's uniform, cap and these boots clomping around the wards all night. Many staff came and went without ever knowing her real name.' Unfortunately Bootsy had the habit of falling fast asleep when she sat down to talk to the nurses. She would be talking and just drop off. She would wake ten minutes or half an hour later and resume her conversation as if she had been awake the whole time, or would say; 'I nearly nodded off then!' She could, on occasions, nod off for up to an hour. The nurses would creep off to do their work, but did not need to be too quiet. She would then come on to the ward with her lovely sheepish grin, and say, 'I must have dropped off for a few minutes.' As Audrey said, 'We respected her though. If we did something wrong, she would stand up for us against the other sisters and even Matron. When there was a crisis she would be there, supporting, advising and giving us confidence. If need be she would roll her sleeves up and pitch right in.'

On June Ardern's very first night in nursing, she was just about to go off duty when she saw an elderly patient coming along the corridor to the top of the stairs, carrying two bulging carrier bags – her worldly possessions. Very unsteady on her feet, she teetered at the top of the stairs. Before June could do anything she tumbled down, and landed at her feet. There was a rush of staff from every direction. Never was she so glad to see someone calmly take over the situation – it was Bootsy. She instantly took control, aware of the needs of the patient and the procedures to follow, and did not forget time for the petrified nurse. When June returned (somewhat apprehensively) the following night she found that the patient had fractured her skull.

On his first night shift and on a medical ward Reg Commander worked with a man called Ginger, also a former regular army man, who was always smiling. His favourite adjective, automatically applied to everything, was 'cowing'. There would be the 'cowing sister', the 'cowing nurses' and the 'cowing patients', all pronounced in a benevolent fashion and accompanied by his cheeky grin. On their third night the ward had one of its quieter nights. By midnight all the work was done and they went to rest by the open fire. 'Have a kip,' said Ginger. 'I'll keep watch. I never sleep. I used to have thirty-six hour shifts doing sentry duty on the cowing North-west Frontier.'

'I thanked him and settled down,' said Reg, 'only to be wakened shortly after by a weird noise; it was Ginger snoring. It seems that the cowing North-western Frontier must have held more dangers to keep him awake than the threat of Night Sister. Not for me though, I never fell asleep again.'

Because friends from the same 'set' could be on night duty together there were often opportunities for fun. On duty at the Royal Masonic Hospital there was one nurse who was particularly uneasy about being left in charge of a ward. Liz Carter and her friends decided to play a prank on her. They stuffed a pair of pyjamas with towels and for a head they fastened on a Guy Fawkes mask. Creeping down to the ward they laid the 'body' with its head in the kitchen oven. Collecting at a window overseeing the kitchen, they phoned the ward and said, 'Check the kitchen, it looks as if one of your patients has his head in the oven.' The nurse scurried along in a panic to be momentarily confronted with the 'body'. Checking and finding out what it was, she looked out of the window to see a group of her hysterical colleagues peering down on her.

These same nurses would buy sweets with soft fruit centres, suck the centres out with a syringe and fill them with frusemide (a diuretic). They would then offer them to the night sister in the hope that she was somewhat inconvenienced and thus reduce the number of visits to the wards. They were never quite sure if it worked but it was all part of the fun of night duty. Another prank was to fill a rubber surgical glove with water and place a stone in it. They would then tie a string to the glove, lower it down to a window where one of their friends was and swing it so that it tapped on the window. Later, when she was a night sister herself, Liz Carter had learned all the tricks.

On her first night on night duty at the London Hospital, Avril Vincent was working near the entrance to the ward when a porter entered pushing a patient on a trolley. The hospital was in the middle of a large Jewish community. The patient was very Jewish looking and was wringing his hands and muttering in what Avril thought was Hebrew. To her astonishment the porter started to hit him around the head. She immediately went to the patient's defence, only to be met by two laughing medical students. That was her initiation to night duty.

When they were tired, night duty nurses could also get very giggly.

Audrey Phillips had many such nights. Once, there was a patient who was on a blood transfusion, and it needed changing.

We did all the usual cross-checking with the notes and the blood and prepared to do the change. The other nurse said, 'Clamp the tube.' I did. Unfortunately in my tired state I did it with my scissors, not the forceps. Well, you can imagine it, there was blood everywhere and to make matters worse we started giggling and we could not stop. The patient was unharmed, in fact slept through the whole thing. Fortunately it was the emptying bottle so by the time we recovered ourselves it was not too bad.

They spent the rest of the night laughing at everything, as one does when mirth strikes.

She was on an orthopaedic ward where patients were kept in bed on traction. 'One night,' she remembers, 'we had given this lady a sedative with an analgesic and this adversely affected her. She was lying in bed seeing "little people" everywhere. "Look, look, there they go, after them!" She demanded. Well you can imagine, we ended up under the bed, incapable of moving.'

In psychiatric hospitals it was very important to stay awake, for the safety of both the patients and the staff. Eddie Dolling explained:

On night duty we had to 'key in' every quarter of an hour. To do this there was a box at the end of the dormitory that the nurse put his pass-key in and turned a click at a time. This was carried out every quarter of an hour the whole night. You could not cheat, as you never knew when the night superintendent would appear. There were usually two of us so we still managed to have a little shut-eye.

There was also time for mischief in this area of nursing. Ian Gibbs of the One Manor Hospital, Salisbury, remembers:

One of the tricks we played was for a nurse to put on a night-shirt and run past the night charge nurse and 'escape' out of one of the doors. He had no option but to chase the supposed patient but we had already tied his shoelaces together while he was supposed to be awake. What could he say?

Another joke was played at almost all hospitals when the nurses knew a body was to be transferred to the mortuary, said Ian:

One of us would get down there quickly and lie on a table under a sheet. When the nurses arrived, whoever it was on the table would then sit up with the sheet still on them. Or we would tell a nurse that a relative had arrived and could he take them to the mortuary. Before he escorted anyone the nurse would first go down to the mortuary and check the body. Of course it would be a member of staff he would find on the table and when he looked under the sheet the 'body' would either wink or speak and scare the life out of him. It all sounds infantile now but in mental hospitals at that time you needed an outlet.

Night should also have been a time for the patients to relax. Wendy Carson was working on a male orthopaedic ward and as usual there were many younger men. It was big fight night, Rocky Marciano versus Don Cockell, being broadcast from the USA, and due to start at 2.00 a.m.

Somehow the patients all managed to stay awake and keep me busy helping them with headphones and making cups of tea. Night Sister came to make her round and gave me a long lecture because so many of the patients were awake, and of course it was my fault. I explained the situation but it made no difference, 'What nonsense,' she said, 'Tell them to turn the radio off and get to sleep.' I told her that lying around in traction all day they were getting plenty of rest and that it must get very boring and this was probably good for them. I suggested to night sister that she should go round and tell them. She did, and nearly had a riot on her hands.

She left the ward rather hurriedly and did not mention it on her morning round.

One night a member of the nursing staff died. She was in her chair, and looked as though she was asleep. The night sister went over to her and said, 'Are you sleeping nurse?' She did not respond, and when the sister put her hand on her she instantly realized that she was dead. The matron, the doctor and the police were all called. The following morning the matron returned to talk to the night nurses and offered each of them sleeping tablets. They were not individually prescribed by a doctor and one can therefore only presume that the matron and the doctor used their own authority to get them from the pharmacy.

Of course there are numerous accounts of ghostly apparitions on night duty, many of them quite convincing. These range from unaccountable changes in temperature and atmosphere to encounters with former nursing staff and patients. Nurses tell of feeling a presence and actually being guided to a bed where a patient had become unconscious, of staff falling asleep and being gently woken, and sisters in grey wandering corridors and wards. At one hospital a mother who had committed suicide was said to be still wandering through the hospital looking for her child, who had died on the children's ward at the hospital. At another hospital a ward sister who had spent her life at the hospital and died on duty was reported to appear on the ward at night. Almost always these are benign experiences although there are reports of poltergeists creating mischief. These stories are exacerbated of course by nurses putting a sheet over themselves and quietly appearing on a ward to scare the life out of their colleagues.

Night duty can be very stressful. Wendy Wild is still unhappy about an incident when one of her young staff nurses lost her father.

She had a nice close family, her mother was obviously young herself. She came back to work after a very short time and she was due on night duty. She came to me and requested not to be put on night duty. I said I would relook at this and gave her another option. The other staff nurses said, 'What on earth did you let her get away with that for, it now means changing with someone else. We have had our own problems and had to get on with it.' Unfortunately, I went against that intuitive feeling, on what I had decided. So I spoke to the nurse and told her that she would have to get on with the night duty. It nearly destroyed her. She was up all night and not sleeping in the daytime. She said to me afterwards that she would look at the older patients with chest pains and heart attacks and think, why are you alive and my young dad is dead? I deeply regretted the decision I had made and I felt I really let her down. My intuition told me what I should have done but my inexperience let me down. I would not repeat that mistake now. I just know that the sister I modelled myself on would not have changed her decision.

Daphne Fallows was the sole night sister in 1958 at the country branch of St Thomas's Hospital at Hydestile, near Godalming. There were some huts for adults, one children's ward, one small theatre and a small accident area. There was little external lighting, and Daphne had to walk from hut to hut up a covered walkway with a torch. On call at night was a junior houseman who was courting one of the nurses, something that would normally be frowned upon. The two of them thought that they were keeping it a great secret from the other staff.

I like to think I was quite kind. When I saw him going into the ward I would give them twenty minutes or so by going to another ward. This would put the ward sequence out but the staff would always know I was on my way because I had to use a torch. He came to me one night and asked, 'Can I talk to you?' He thanked me, and said that they knew very well that I had been aware of their courtship and that they wanted me to be the first to know that she had just accepted his proposal.

Now a volunteer at the Florence Nightingale Museum at St Thomas's Hospital, Daphne was on duty with a younger volunteer when a rather elderly lady came in and said to her, 'I know you from when I was a patient at Hydestile, you were night sister. I was very upset and you took me to your office for a cup of tea and talked to me. You have not changed at all.'

'Then it dawned on me,' Daphne recalled. 'I could not remember her name but even now I could tell you the bed she was in, her diagnosis and treatment!' The young volunteer asked Daphne when this was. When she said 1958, the girl replied, 'My goodness my mother was not even born then!'

18   A Proud Heritage

Despite our financial and economic anxieties, we are still able to
do the most civilized thing in the world – put the welfare of the
sick in front of every other consideration.

> Aneurin Bevan on the new National Health Service,
> 9 February 1948

Florence Nightingale recognized 150 years ago that many patients,
and particularly the elderly, were susceptible to infection through
illness or social conditions before being admitted to hospital. From
her experience at Scutari Hospital in the Crimea, she also learned
that a patient's physical condition could deteriorate with poor dietary
intake or infection through poor hygiene standards, and that one or
both of these increased the morbidity and mortality on the wards. At
the very least these factors would further complicate an illness,
reduce the patient's wound-healing abilities and delay recovery. She
made a decision that strong nurse leadership in the form of a matron,
backed up at ward level by sisters, would be the key to protecting
patients from these and other threats to their health. The sisters who
were appointed to these positions were people who could lead on
good practice and develop care based around the patients' needs.

It was a hierarchical system that also provided clear lines of
accountability. From the most junior person in any area of the hospital to the most senior, everyone was directly accountable to someone.
When a new nurse entered the profession she knew immediately who
her senior was and respected that position – not always the person
but certainly the position. As her career progressed she would be
clearly accountable to someone in a higher position until she reached
the post of matron and then she would be directly accountable to a

board of governors. Accountability for errors in practice is and always has been the responsibility of the individual nurse.

On the ward, the sister was the clearly identified person in charge. Patients, visitors, medical staff, porters and domestic staff knew this; no one would enter a ward without reporting to the sister first. In this position she was the centre of knowledge, so she could be relied upon for information about any of the patients on her ward, and for orchestrating the care around them. All services in the ward were regulated and controlled by her. The willingness of sister to pass her knowledge on has always been central to the development of nursing.

Since it was introduced in 1948 the National Health Service has been a caring organization that has provided an uninterrupted service to millions of its patients. But it requires a huge budget to fund the ever-increasing demands placed on it and responsible management to prioritize these demands. Devising measures and targets for hospital numbers are one thing, devising measures and targets for care around the patient is another. The traditional sister did not have such concerns; she had inherited what she considered were high standards of care and she was the keeper and bestower of these standards to generations of nurses – standards unchallenged throughout the world. 'I think we had the best of it,' said one nurse. 'The 1950s and 1960s were the heyday of nursing, it was all so exciting, you felt you were on the crest of something really good. The NHS was still new and we felt, as nurses, that we were instrumental in shaping it. We did have some influence and we were proud to be nurses.'

With advances in the medical treatment of patients inevitably came demands for more beds and more money to finance these developments. Once the demands started to accelerate a different approach to managing this change had to be introduced. Along with these accelerated service demands society was also changing. The societal trends associated with this change were out of step with the demands of a traditional hierarchical system. Where a girl in the 1950s would think nothing of working the long hours demanded at that time, this work load had no place at the end of the twentieth century. This does not mean that people are less caring; there are endless examples of selfless giving to others in our society and there always will be. Nursing has always been a route by which people could help others and it will continue to be so. Many of the traditional sisters are now

243

users of the service and speak highly of the advances in treatment and the care from individual nurses. 'I was in hospital for a triple heart bypass operation,' said one. 'I was only in for a few days and this astonished me, compared to what happened in my days of nursing; I could not believe it possible. I could not complain about the nurses, they were hard working and very kind.'

A former tutor commented:

These are exciting times for nursing. As more and more complex conditions are being treated leading to longer life expectancy, individual nurses can now make greater contributions in many clinical areas: endoscopy, respiratory care, diabetes, urology, and now it is suggested anaesthesiology. With this change, nurses are taking over many jobs that were previously those of junior medical staff. As a consequence some of the roles that were those of the junior doctors are being handed down to specialist sisters, taking some sisters away from the ward setting. This is inevitably leading to changes in the way nurses are trained. It used to be that sister tutor and clinical teachers supported the clinical role on the wards by linking theory to practice. At the bedside, the traditional sister would then teach issues of cleanliness, observational skills and clinical practice. The most junior nurse would quickly learn to spot the perils of dust on a locker or a dirty swab on the floor. They would also be able to recognize the signs of a dry mouth or respiratory distress; it was the way we learned.

This led a nurse to say:

Nursing has become more technical, and the health service is treating more patients, also society has higher expectations, but some things should not change. Where our focus was on bed-care – the patient was in for longer periods of time – now the focus is on bed usage and nursing has to adapt to this. But nursing has always adapted to changing demands; after all it coped well with two world wars and the introduction of organ transplants. Nursing has also been hard work, and it always will be. But at the end of the day, the physical and emotional well-being

244

of the patient should always be its priority.

Among the numerous anecdotes collected for this book, there was some envy, but also considerable sympathy with the demands of present-day nursing. The envy was for the shorter working hours, the enhanced remuneration and the freedoms; the sympathy was for the cost of these improvements. Said one former sister:

When I was nursing there was tremendous job satisfaction. Having worked on a surgical ward for many years I found I had great respect for the sister running the ward I was a patient on; she hardly seemed to have time to breathe. The few moments we spoke I found out that she had a family of her own. I thought at the time, with patients in and out in days or even hours, a home and children to look after when the working day is over, how did she manage? If I was needed on the ward I could stay on, but the sister of the ward I was on looked to me like a juggler trying to keep all the balls in the air at the same time, rushing like mad to complete everything before going home. Stress is not new – we were often stressed – but it was not the negative self-destructive thing of today.

One nurse pointed out:

I know the generation of today will look back to our time and think, 'I would not want those days again, all that discipline and long hours, I need my time off, I have too much to do.' But I wonder if they have missed out on the job satisfaction, the comradeship, the teamwork and the laughter of those days. I know it is not nostalgia, not looking through rose-tinted glasses; there are things I would not want back again. But it was the pride we had of belonging to an organization that was respected.

These traditional sisters do not see themselves as icons of perfection, but they feel that their finger was always on the pulse of ward activity. They also saw nursing as a privilege. 'What was so marvellous,' one former sister recalls from 1936, 'was when matron inter-

245

viewed me at St George's Hospital, London, she said, "If I accept you, you must first realize what a privilege it is to wear a nurse's uniform and what a privilege it is to nurse the sick." ' Nurses were always aware of their nursing heritage, not only through the hierarchical system, but also through the wearing of their traditional uniform, belts and buckles. Other occasions were the matron's prize-giving, and her annual ball, all these engendering great pride in nursing, in belonging to 'their' hospital. As one former nurse pointed out, 'We were very proud of how we looked in those days, and we would just die for the strings and bows you got from Matron, you almost burst with the honour of it. I am sure this would not be understood today.'

I realized after the publication of my previous book, *When Matron Ruled*, just how strongly nurses felt about their nursing heritage. Nurses wrote of their disappointment that their hospital or matron was not mentioned. As with this book, it was not possible to include all hospitals. Olga Marshall, a former sister, wrote of her pride at having worked for Miss Lucy Duff Grant, matron of Manchester Royal Infirmary, who was created a dame. Olga recalled:

I wrote to congratulate Miss Duff-Grant and was invited to tea at her Kensington apartment. I arrived to be faced by one of those entry doors that had a call system. I could not get an answer. Fortunately another resident came along and I explained to her who I wished to see. I nearly fell flat on my face when she said, 'Oh. Miss Duff-Grant, what a dear old poppet she is.' With my memory of a tall, well-built, majestic figure oozing dignity and authority, revered and feared by everyone, I nearly exploded. A poppet indeed! Such lack of respect! At the age of ninety-three I still look back on my nursing years with great pride.

Bibliography

Abel-Smith, B., *A History of the Nursing Profession* (Heinmann, 1960)
Clifford, Collette (ed), *QE Nurse 1938–1957* (Brewin Books, 1997)
Coventry, S., *Images of a Nightingale* (Beauclerk Publishing, 1990)
Davies, Celia, *Rewriting Nursing History* (Croom Helm, 1980)
Fox, M.E., *How to Become a Nurse* (The Scientific Press, c. 1925)
Humphry, L., *A Manual of Nursing* (Charles Griffin & Company, 1891)
Hussey, M., *A Memoir by Marmaduke Hussey* (Macmillan, 2002)
Morton, Honor, *How to Become a Nurse* (The Scientific Press, 1895)
Ramsay, Edith, *East London Nursing Society 1868–1968: The History of a Hundred Years* (Beacon Press, 1968)
Rubinstein, David, *Victorian Homes* (David & Charles, 1974)
Webster, Charles, *Aneurin Bevan in the National Health Service* (Wellcome Unit for the History of Medicine, 1991)
Yeo, G., *Nursing at Bart's* (Sutton Publishing, 1995)

Index